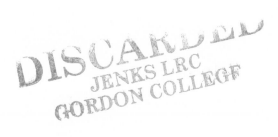

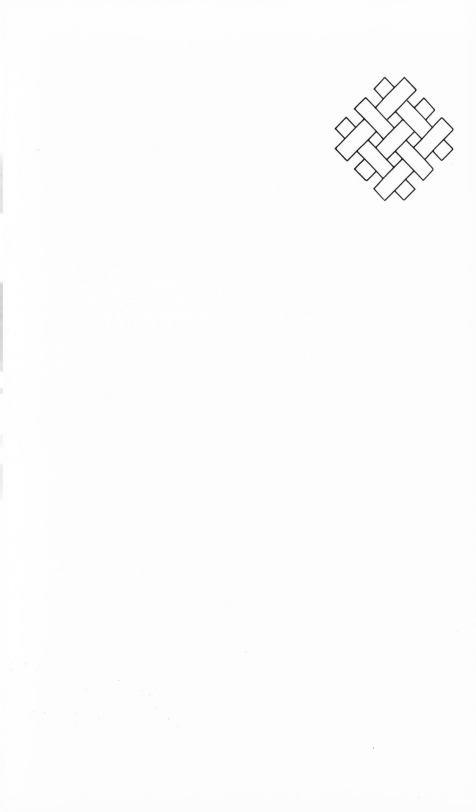

REGIONS OF THE MIND

Brain Research and the Quest for Scientific Certainty

Susan Leigh Star

Stanford University Press
Stanford, California ◊ 1989

Stanford University Press
Stanford, California
© 1989 by the Board of Trustees of the
Leland Stanford Junior University
Printed in the United States of America

CIP data appear at the end of the book

for Fran and Anselm Strauss
beloved friends and teachers

and for my parents, Glenn and Shirley Kippax
with love and respect

Acknowledgments

All scientific work is collective. I have been lucky to conduct this research in a generous and gifted community of scholars. I am especially grateful to Adele Clarke, Joan Fujimura, Elihu Gerson, Anselm Strauss, and Rachel Volberg for their help. Many of the ideas here draw on their work and on discussions with them. Anselm spent many hours with me analyzing and helping me to integrate my findings, and teaching me about the processes and varieties of work. Adele, Joan, and Rachel were good friends, colleagues, and critics. Elihu provided valuable criticism in the early stages of the project. Howard Becker also made many helpful suggestions on chapter drafts.

I would also like to thank the following people for helpful and often extensive comments and discussion of the work presented here: Pauline Bart, the late Herbert Blumer, the late Rue Bucher, Kathy Charmaz, Nan Chico, M. Sue Gerson, Kathleen Gregory Huddleston, James Griesemer, Gail Hornstein, Ruth Hubbard, Bud Hutchins, Bruno Latour, John Law, Ruth Linden, Marilyn Little, Carl Hewitt, Lynda Koolish, Jane Maienschein, Sheryl Ruzek, Ken Schaffner, Lenny Schatzman, Dan Todes, Barry Wellman, and William C. Wimsatt. Wimsatt's work is pivotal to many of the concepts discussed here. I am grateful to Ralph Kellogg for discussion of resources in the history of physiology. Muriel Bell, senior editor at Stanford University Press, added many insights and clarifications.

My respondents for the pilot study graciously allowed me to observe them at work and to interview them. Sigrid Novikoff and Mirto Stone translated the work of Goltz and Panizza, respectively (Appendixes A and B). Ruth Linden provided valuable bibliographic assistance. William Goodenough House, London, provided living accommodations during my stay in London.

I would like to thank the staff of the National Hospital for Nervous Diseases, Queen Square, London (formerly the National Hospital for the Paralysed and Epileptic) for allowing me to read their nineteenth-century patient records. Special thanks are due to John Marshall, then dean, Institute of Neurology; Paula Porter, patients services officer, National Hospital for Nervous Diseases; Gladys Seville, medical records officer; and Iris Royer, Outpatients Department, for their time and assistance.

The following libraries and archives generously made their resources available to me: Thane Medical Library, University College, London, with special thanks for access to Victor Horsley's casebooks; the archives of the Royal Society, London; the library of the Royal College of Physicians, London, with special thanks for access to David Ferrier's unpublished laboratory notebooks; the Wellcome Library for the History of Medicine; and the UCSF collection in the History of Medicine.

Some of the original research for this project was assisted by funds from the University of California, San Francisco. Tremont Research Institute, San Francisco, generously provided organizational resources. A fellowship from La Fondation Fyssen allowed me to study and compare approaches with colleagues at the Centre de sociologie de l'innovation, École des Mines, in France. Sally and Pete Becker kindly allowed me to use their printer. Several aspects of the research were conducted jointly with Tremont and the MIT Artificial Intelligence Lab's Message Passing Semantics Group. This group has used studies of the scientific community as a source of metaphors for building their models of complex, highly parallel decision-making. I am especially grateful to Carl Hewitt for comments and support—and for providing a source of metaphors from computer science for sociological work!

Lynda Koolish deserves special thanks for her support of this project. My husband and friend, Geof Bowker, has been a superb critic and midwife. My parents, Glenn and Shirley Kippax, are continuing sources of inspiration and support.

Finally, I would like to thank Lucien Schneider for teaching me to play twenty questions.

Preface

It was a cold, gray London morning in 1875. A bell rang repeatedly inside the National Hospital at Queen Square, slowly rousing the night porter/guard who lay slumbering in his chair near the back ward. The guard opened the door to see two men, one a disgruntled fellow of middle age, hat pulled down over his eyes against the cold, supporting another who slumped against him, eyes closed.

"This here's the fits hospital, right?" said the upright one. Upon hearing the affirmative, he shook the fellow leaning against him and attempted to push him into the arms of the night attendant. "Here, what's this about?" said the surprised porter. The arms of the limp man had been bound to his sides with a rough rope. Suspecting foul play, the porter began to explain that this was no general hospital or emergency ward, but that patients could only be admitted here with the approval of a patron, with the diagnosis of nervous disease, paralysis, or epilepsy.

"The stationmaster give me the fare to bring this poor bloke over here, that's all I know," said the first man, evidently a cab driver. "He can't talk, can't walk, and shakes all over every five minutes. Got shipped down here from somewhere out in Yorkshire, the man at the station said. Folks didn't know what else to do." There was no sign of recognition or affirmation from the bound man. The porter reached out and fingered a label that had been attached to the rope on the man's body, a sort of large, crude mailing label. In rough handwriting were simply the words, "Fits Hospital, London."

Suddenly the bound man began to shake, wrenching from the cabbie's grasp, and fell to the ground. The reason for the ropes became apparent as he flailed from side to side, arms straining against them. The cabbie and the night porter dragged him across the threshold.

They put pillows around him so that he would not hurt himself, and they placed a bit of cotton wadding under his tongue.

The man could neither speak nor walk, and between seizures he lay apathetically in the back ward for several days. Attendants administered potassium bromide and held him down when the seizures came. Finally, John Hughlings Jackson, the physician to the hospital and an expert on epilepsy, made his weekly visit. The patient had been quiet for hours, resting docilely, looking blankly at the ceiling. As Jackson was making his rounds, however, a seizure began. Jackson was quickly summoned to the bedside. He observed the sequence of spasms, which began in the man's left-hand fingers, moved up the arm, and gradually involved the whole body.

Jackson diagnosed a tumor with a localized origin in the right temporal lobe of the brain, and he hypothesized that the tumor was causing the seizures to occur in a specific location and sequence. More potassium bromide, electrotherapy, hydrotherapy, and massage were prescribed.

Subsequent seizures were recorded in detail by the night porters and day attendants as they attempted to replicate Jackson's observations about the origin of the spasms, duration of seizures, and severity of spasm. The patient did not respond to the bromide, and both electrotherapy and massage frequently brought on seizures, so the attendants tried to make these therapies as short and infrequent as possible. The porters tried to note the details of the seizures, but it was difficult. Often the patient would begin twitching or flailing about in the middle of the night. Sleepy attendants would rush in with a candle and make sure the patient came to no harm. The light and noise wakened other patients in the ward, and calming the disruption took some time. Afterwards, the attendants would fill out detailed "fits sheets" that recorded observations of each seizure including sequence, muscles involved, and where the twitching started.

After three months the unidentified patient suddenly went into a coma and died. With no relatives in the picture, a rare opportunity for a leisurely autopsy was afforded to Jackson and the hospital staff. Jackson's thesis was that the tumor had destroyed parts of the speech and motor areas, causing the inability to speak and the paralysis. The seizures had come from what he called the "discharging" properties of the tumor, which animated the muscles. During the autopsy a large tumor was found, and it partially impinged on the areas Jackson had predicted.

Thus, from analysis of the disordered behavior and presumably disordered mental capacities of the patient, Jackson and the other researchers at the National Hospital for the Paralysed and Epileptic, Queen Square, London, searched for and found the physical areas they thought caused the behavior. They were able, on this occasion, to open up the mysterious twitching "package" presented at their doorstep and point to what they believed to be a juncture between the mind and the brain.

Meanwhile, one day shortly after Mr. X died, in a dimly lit laboratory down the street, David Ferrier was performing his second operation of the day on the brain of a macaque monkey. The first animal had died earlier that afternoon from an overdose of chloroform; Ferrier fervently hoped that this one would live long enough for him to observe the effects of the lesion he was making in the brain. His goal was to produce a lesion in the same area as Jackson's patient had had the brain tumor. If the monkey stopped walking or moving, he and Jackson could claim further evidence for the link between motor activity and a certain area of the brain.

Ferrier's worries were many: the monkeys were expensive;[1] his budget was limited; he could not afford to be away from patients for long; and the antivivisectionist movement was growing stronger and more politically powerful (French 1975). If he could only get positive results before they moved to close down his laboratory! His practice was growing as a result of fame from his experiments, yet he got no released time or pay to do physiological research, still considered a sort of hobby in English medical circles.

It had been a long week. Yesterday's experimental subject, a large female macaque, had been most recalcitrant. She had run away from Ferrier, snarled, and knocked the electrodes from his hands when he had tried to apply the galvanic current to her brain to test her muscle movements.

Even when experiments went smoothly, it was often hard to tell exactly which functions had been impaired by the surgical lesions or which parts of the brain were responding to current. Were the limbs twitching, or moving under the electrical stimulus? Was the paralysis from impairment of an area of the brain, or was it shock from the operation itself? Ferrier often could not be sure.

Finally, the monkey began to come out of the anesthesia. Ferrier bandaged up the head wound from the operation, then sat down wearily and waited for the animal to come to consciousness. He lit a gas burner at one end of the room and made a pot of strong tea.

Several hours later, the monkey irritably clung to the hot water pipes, the only source of heat in the cold basement laboratory. Ferrier gave the animal a saucer of tea and noted that she was able to drink it. Like the night attendant in the hospital, he tried to jot down an accurate record of the symptoms exhibited by his subject, including twitches and epileptic seizures. At night's end, Ferrier and the monkey stared at one another across the lab, drinking their respective cups of tea.

Later, Ferrier would write up his results in *The Functions of the Brain*, a book widely circulated and reviewed in medical circles in Europe and the United States.[2] There he would claim that he had helped to find the elusive mind/brain connection. A second package had been opened. Now the two contents could be joined to make and strengthen a third: the theory of localization of function.

The circumstances described here in both situations are composites, drawn together to convey a vivid description of the work situations faced by these scientists.[3] Their aim was to discover the nature of brain functions, especially the link between brain and behavior.

An instructor in my first sociology class remarked that beginning sociology students are always amazed by the number and variety of breakdowns, mistakes, and incongruities in the field sites they choose to study. "What never strikes them at first," he chuckled, "is that what is really amazing is that there should be *any* order, any regularity there in all that chaos! Now *that's* what's really amazing!"[4]

The remarkable regularity investigated by this book is the development, late in the nineteenth century, of an extremely successful theory about the nature of the brain. The theory was successful because it was both plastic and many-rooted. Its roots and its plastic nature were created by the work and concerns of a group of scientists, administrators, patients, and social reformers. This is the story of that work, including the formidable practical problems and uncertainties these people faced and the role played by their institutions, professions, and political enmities. It is also the story of how perspectives evolve and how people come to believe what they do about nature, based on how, and under what conditions, they do work.

Contents

ONE	Studying Scientific Work	I
TWO	The Institutional Contexts of Localization Research	38
THREE	Uncertainty and Scientific Work	62
FOUR	Triangulating Clinical and Basic Research	96
FIVE	The Debate About Cerebral Localization	118
SIX	The Mind/Brain Problem: Parallelism and Localization	155
SEVEN	The Legacy of Localizationism	175
	Appendixes	199
	Notes	233
	References Cited	241
	Indexes	271

Regions of the Mind

I am neither a universaliser nor a localiser. . . . In consequence I have been attacked as a universaliser and also as a localiser. But I do not remember that the view I really hold as to localisation has ever been referred to. If it is, it will very likely be supposed to be a fusion of, or a compromise betwixt, recent doctrines.   —John Hughlings Jackson (1932e: 35)

The structure and working of the brain had been laid bare, and the stupendous fact had been established that to each of the cerebral hemispheres were allotted functions distinct and separate. These enthusiasts, pursuing their investigations under discouraging conditions with an untiring patience which invested their intelligence with genius, demonstrated that every individual portion of the seemingly homogeneous organ was allotted its own particular task, and in response to the probing interrogations of science every fibre and filament of the complex structure yielded up the secret of its being.
—Burford Rawlings, administrator,
National Hospital for the Paralysed and Epileptic,
in the nineteenth century (Rawlings 1913)

As to them blooming doctors, we teach 'em a lot, I know. Lor! how they do jaw about our insides to them blokes as sits and looks on.   —Patient, National Hospital for
the Paralysed and Epileptic, in the
nineteenth century (Rawlings 1913)

Studying Scientific Work

> There are in the human mind a group of faculties and in the brain
> groups of convolutions, and the facts assembled by science so far al-
> low to state, as I said before, that the great regions of the mind cor-
> respond to the great regions of the brain.
> —Paul Broca, 1861 (quoted in von Bonin 1950: 57)

This is a book about scientific work. Like any form of
practice, science is at once boring and dramatic, uncertain and routine, amateur and professional. Yet because science has been treated
as a special kind of activity by so many scholars, for so long, its analysis as work per se has been largely neglected.

Imagine a study of Christian religious work, conducted by a
scholar in, say, the Middle Ages in Europe. The study outlines the
process by which priests and nuns choose careers; details the fights
for resources between various monasteries and abbeys; describes the
impact of publishing technology on the dissemination of theology;
explains how servants help keep the churches clean and orderly, and
so on. Such a study would be of great interest to social scientists comparing work organization in various settings. It might illuminate
some of the infrastructure of belief and power in medieval Christian
populations; it might also prove useful for historical institutional
comparison as the church developed in later years. But by its very position as a study of work, and not as a work of true belief, the author
of the study is thought to call into question the very tenets of faith.
Although it is true that, logically, such a study could proceed in tandem with, or even independent of, specific articles of faith, in a theo-
cratic society a study of the mundane and menial aspects of religious
work is heretical.

Such is the case with the sociology of science in the 1980's. It is impossible to write a book about scientific work without calling into question the fundamental tenets of the belief in science. If scientists are "merely workers," not highly trained instruments illuminating the truth resident in nature, then where does truth reside? If their work is revealed as uncertain, error-prone, simplified, or biased, then what can we trust? Is there progress in science, or merely directionless change?

In order to answer these questions sociologically, it has been necessary for me to write a book that falls between disciplinary cracks and tackles these questions on their own terms. These are questions that have traditionally fallen under the purview of philosophy and the history of science. Philosophers, historians, and scientists themselves have debated them at length, often using one another's work to do so. But with rare exceptions, and until the past few years, practice has remained immune to analysis.

Everyone agrees that science is an important institution. Why then have there been so few studies of scientific work? One explanation is that it is difficult to study science as practice. First, the language of a science must be learned (a substantial investment of time); the above-mentioned questions must be resolved well enough to be able to proceed; and some tractable scientists, alive or dead, must be found to study. Second, it is intimidating to study an institution with so many active believers who have control over one's own career and fate, and who in turn are believed by all of one's colleagues. It is one thing to study prostitutes or addicts at some remove from the university, or to study a cult with few adherents. It is another to study the practice of what is, in fact, the dominant religion of one's own place of work. This is difficult not only as a risk in terms of one's career (that remains to be seen for this current generation of sociologists of science), but also as a risk emotionally and philosophically. Studying science exposes all the hard questions about nature, values, positivism, truth, and beauty. And it is not the case that all believers welcome such questions if the answers they provoke are unorthodox.

In spite of the difficulties, however, studying scientific practice is exciting and liberating. In the conduct of scientific work lies a new kind of answer to the old philosophical and historical questions about truth and change. That is what this book is about.

Although this book is a study of a group of brain researchers, its application is more general than the history of physiology or medicine. What is the nature of scientific change? I hope to provide a model here for understanding such change as communal, complex, historical, and situated in practice and work organization. One does not have to be interested in brain research per se to be interested in the nature of change and practice in science, or indeed in any complex organization.

I come from an intellectual tradition, American symbolic interactionist sociology, which tends to stress the everyday ways in which people are alike (Blumer 1969; Hughes 1971a). Scientists—like priests, bus drivers, parents, or criminals—work. As with all work, there are routines and emergencies, organizational hierarchies and power relations, uncertainties and conflicts. By attempting in this volume to discuss scientists as workers, it is not my intent to create an exposé of science, to prove that it "isn't really real." On the contrary, I believe that understanding work practices in science gives us a new understanding of the sturdiness of scientific findings. People create meaning when they undertake joint action. Scientific meaning—truth, or theories, or facts—is the result of innumerable encounters, actions, and situations (see Fujimura, Star, and Gerson 1987).[1]

Localizationist Brain Research: General Background

Early in the 1870's a handful of medical researchers, primarily British, envisioned a map of the brain that would match each mental function with a single physical area. Many of these researchers were based at the National Hospital for the Paralysed and Epileptic, Queen Square, London (now the National Hospital for Nervous Diseases). They promised that such a map would solve an array of medical puzzles, including the etiology and physical basis of epilepsy, aphasia, brain tumors, stroke, syphilis, and tuberculosis. The mappers were also bidding to answer some of the most hotly debated questions in philosophy, theology, physiology, and psychology: the nature of the relationship between the brain and the "mind" (Danziger 1982) and whether there could be a biological explanation for complex human behaviors.

Between 1870 and 1906, these researchers faced constant, severe uncertainties, most of which were never resolved. Many of the medical and scientific community ridiculed their initial mapping efforts as neophrenology. But by 1906, with the publication of Charles Scott Sherrington's *The Integrative Action of the Nervous System*, the map and its underlying premises had become an unquestioned fact in the medical and physiological work of the West. How these researchers moved from ridicule to prominence is a long and complex story; this book explores several aspects of it.

Brain research has a long and chaotic history. From Aristotle to the present, its hallmarks have been bitter debate, disagreement, and confusion in the face of enormous complexity. Broadly speaking, two classes of theory have been accepted at different times and places: localization theories and diffusion theories (Swazey 1970).

Localization theories hold that the brain (especially the cerebral hemispheres) is composed of distinct parts, each with its sovereign function. The familiar term "speech area" reflects this view. Diffusion theories hold that the brain operates holistically, without separation of parts or a pointillist division of labor. Barbara Tizard (1959: 132) noted that, historically, "a swing of the pendulum tends to occur between these two positions. At one period the majority of informed opinion holds a localization theory, but a generation later this tends to be considered distinctly unorthodox." Judith Swazey (1969) reports a similar swing between theories of "action propre" and "action commune" in the brain research community.

Phrenology, popular from the end of the eighteenth century until about 1830, is perhaps the best known example of a localizationist theory. Phrenologists held that a person's character could be "read" through the bumps on the skull. Each bump represented a different faculty or trait (Shapin 1979). Between 1840 and 1860 (after phrenology had become scientifically unfashionable), dominant scientific theories of brain function became diffusionist. The influential work of the French physiologist Pierre Flourens had demonstrated that the cerebral hemispheres did not have areas associated with particular functions. His primary experimental animals had been pigeons; he generalized these animal findings to human brains. He believed the hemispheres to be insensible to stimulation and to operate as indivisible wholes (Walker 1957).[2]

During the 1860's a strong interest in localization of function in the cerebral hemispheres began to develop among Western medical researchers. Paul Broca, in France, demonstrated his famous eponymous speech area in 1861. One of his patients died who had suffered severely impaired speech ability. Autopsy showed a softening of the brain in the third frontal convolution (Broca 1861, 1863). Amid great controversy, Broca publicized this finding and claimed broad implications for the brain as a whole (Riese 1977: 68; Schiller 1979). This idea became a mandate and program for subsequent researchers.

Meanwhile, in England, John Hughlings Jackson was working with epileptic patients, attempting to account for the bewildering array of symptoms they exhibited. Jackson was heavily influenced by the philosopher Herbert Spencer. He attempted to apply Spencer's theories of evolution and dissolution of society directly to the nervous system (see, for example, Jackson 1932a, 1932e). He focused on the progression of symptoms in epilepsy. By the early 1870's he had begun to associate them with specific parts of the brain and to integrate them into a theoretical model.

In 1870 brain research reached a turning point. Two German investigators, Gustav Fritsch and Eduard Hitzig (1950 [1870]), discovered that electrical stimulation applied to various areas of an animal's cortex (cerebral hemispheres) would produce *specific* muscle reactions. English medical experimenters immediately seized on the implications of this research. Efforts to tie together reflex physiology, clinical work with epileptics and aphasics, and electrical stimulation experiments got seriously under way at this point (Jefferson 1955; Brazier 1959; Spillane 1981). Among those who contributed significantly to these efforts was David Ferrier, later a colleague of Jackson's at Queen Square. He began his physiological experiments in the early 1870's (Ferrier 1873).

A Historical Puzzle

A striking sociological and historical puzzle sparked this research. In the 1860's the physician Charles-Edouard Brown-Séquard developed a model of the brain based on dynamic and inhibiting forces. He held that multiple brain and nervous system regions were responsible, in a distributed fashion, for the same functions. This diffusionist view would today be considered a holistic view of the mind/body relationship, particularly with regard to nervous function and epilepsy (Brown-Séquard 1860, 1873a). Brown-Séquard was in fact a vociferous critic of the idea of localization of function. From the early 1870's until his death in 1894, he published a series of scathing critiques of localizationism and pursued a course of research designed to refute its findings. In return for this, he was ridiculed and ostracized by localizationists, and his findings were alternately denied and ignored by them.

Yet a gradual and startling evolution occurred in the 30 years before his death. Much of the evidence cited by Brown-Séquard (and other diffusionists) to argue against localization was in the form of anomalies—results counter to localizationist predictions. The central anomaly was that of *inconstant correlation*. Simply, this occurred whenever the relationship between brain area and function did not hold—for instance, if a patient had a tumor on the left side of the brain in the "speech area," yet was able to speak. Brown-Séquard experimentally produced lesions and tried to demonstrate that no dysfunction followed. Where dysfunctions had occurred in patients, or did occur in the experiments, he explained them by reference to the dynamics of certain forces circulating throughout the body.

By the turn of the century, most localizationists had recognized the anomaly of inconstant correlation as a problem for their theory. Yet they did not turn to diffusionism as an alternative; instead, they crafted localizationist explanations for the phenomena. Perhaps, they said, there were *many* centers of localized function that could substitute for each other in the event of failure of one of them. Perhaps each "center" held a part of the total function, and the parts must be combined before action could take place. Perhaps people could under some conditions develop new centers, which would explain the puzzle of recovery of function in the presence of a permanently damaged or removed "center."

As noted above, Sherrington—the direct inheritor of the Queen Square localizationist enterprise—published his major work, *The Integrative Action of the Nervous System*, in 1906. It was dedicated to Ferrier, the famous localizationist and bitter enemy of Brown-Séquard (Ferrier 1876). Sherrington's model of the brain featured inhibition, the flow of nervous information, and, most important, coordination of "decentralized centers." The model was theoretically indistinguishable in most significant ways from Brown-Séquard's. In the comparison of Brown-Séquard and Sherrington we have the central puzzle: if the two models are structurally and logically so similar, why the conflict? Why did localization of function succeed as distinct from more diffusionist models? Were the tenets of diffusionism ignored by localizationists, or were they absorbed into localizationist neurophysiology? How? The answer lies not in the comparison of ideas, but in the social history of work.

Sherrington's techniques and sponsorship came from localizationist physiology. Many of his failures to establish one-to-one correlations between brain areas and behavior had already been experienced by earlier localizationists. Sherrington's work assimilated and synthesized many of these persistent anomalies as minor or insignificant exceptions in the face of a meta-theory of reflexes and actions. Instead of being a challenge to the basic tenets of localization, his model was hailed as its major, if not crowning, achievement.

The argument of this book is that because the theory of localization of function was embedded in, and indistinguishable from, scientific practice, it was not the logical evolution of the theory that was compelling to practitioners, but rather the way their work was structured. By understanding the way the work was organized, we can find the only possible solution to the puzzle.

Sherrington's findings followed several decades of research in which localizationists had struggled to account for anomalous findings within their model. The picture I present in this book is one of complex assimilation of experimental and clinical mismatches between brain region and function. The conditions of assimilation were the result of commitments to ways of working and political alliances developed in the course of localizationist inquiry.

Some historians have found puzzling the sequence of events leading to the "acceptance" of Sherrington's work as part of localization theory. For example, the historian of physiology F. M. R. Walshe remarked that the generation following the classic localizationist studies followed the "plan" of the cortex as originally laid out, despite countervailing evidence from Sherrington. Sherrington posited that functional organization, not simply location, was crucial to the explanation of theretofore anomalous data from localization experiments. Walshe exclaimed over the paradox: it was striking that Sherrington's findings should have been interpreted as evidence for localization of function, "for surely they were the heaviest blow this theory had so far received" (1947: 8). Walshe also found that successive experimental localizationist studies of the cortex could not account for the anomalies that Sherrington claimed as discoveries.

Andrew Peacock (1982) cogently argues that, although Sherrington's work logically pointed to a diffusionist model for behavior and especially to higher cognitive functions, neurophysiologists' institutional ties to localization prevented them from adopting this point of view. Instead, they renegotiated the significance of the failure of localizationist experiments to fit the basic assumptions of localization. This was neither a short nor a simple process. The puzzle I posed above has no simple logical answer, but rather a complex historical one.

From the outset of their work, the scientists under study here wagered their scientific reputations on—and invested substantial resources in—producing functional, localized maps of the brain. Their clinical practices as physicians flourished and in large part depended on their scientific successes in this realm.* They rendered localization convincing through a number of strategies. They entrained the resources of medical professionalization in the service of the theory. They gained ownership of the means of knowledge production and distribution (such as journals, hospital practices, and teaching posts) and screened out opposing points of view from print and employment. They were able to link a successful clinical program with the model; this program was created via experimentation on a population of desperate patients. The localizationists also united against common enemies with powerful scientists from other fields, including Charles Darwin and Thomas Henry Huxley.

*British terminology and distinctions between types of medical jobs can be confusing. I use the following terms: "doctors" is generic, referring to medical personnel including surgeons and house and consulting physicians. Surgeons were doctors who performed operations; physicians diagnosed and consulted. Neurologists were physicians. The lines of work I describe here are not necessarily strictly divided by personnel. For example, physiological experiments and pathological work were done by both surgeons and physicians. For the sake of simplicity I refer to physiologists and pathologists as separate. Since the analysis is based on tasks, not persons, this should present no analytic problems (Walshe 1957; Riese 1959).

The commitment of this group of researchers to a model of cerebral function that would locate behaviors in a physical substratum began at a time of professional upheaval. In medicine, physiology, and other areas of science that touched on the "mind" or "soul," there were heated debates about human nature, the limits of science, and the notion of progress. The scientific stake in demonstrating a physical basis of mind was extraordinarily high in terms of the audiences affected and the resources in jeopardy.

The idea of a physical substratum for behaviors that most contemporary researchers would call mental did not, however, originate in the 1860's. It had complex multiple roots in several social and philosophical traditions. Our commonplace designation of Cartesian dualism refers to Descartes's exposition of the brain/soul relationship. This is often cited as the origin of modern localizationist thought— Descartes thought the two domains came together in the pineal gland. Other writers have traced the mind/body/soul/brain tangle to Aristotle or even to the evolution of consciousness itself.

But whatever the roots of Cartesian dualism and psychophysical parallelism, it was one of the enduring assumptions that informed and legitimated localization theory. These assumptions were embodied in a set of approaches to methods of physiological investigation and to the relationship between the anatomy of the nervous system (structure) and physiology (process). These ideas informed not only localization research but research in many other lines of work as well. In localization research they took the following, often tacit, forms:

1. Physical structures carry or conduct mental functions in the same way that electrical power lines conduct electrical current (put another way, anatomy is a substratum for thought).

2. The mind is contained in the individual brain, especially in the cerebral hemispheres.

3. The mind is divisible into a hierarchically ordered nervous system.

4. The mind/brain relationship can be investigated by removing or deleting parts of the anatomy that perform the function, and then observing changes in behavior. I call this "the logic of deletion."

These assumptions became both production technology and product for localization theory. That is, they were used to rationalize and justify the use of certain methods, the choice of questions, and research directions. And, as the research enterprise itself became a going concern, attracting clients, personnel, and financial support, it legitimated the assumptions, imbuing them with a sense of inevitability and naturalness.

Finding Sources of Evidence for Localization

Scientists from several lines of work became involved in building localization theory. These included neurology, surgery, pathology, and physiology.

Neurologists classified and located nervous diseases, tested, diagnosed, and examined patients, wrote up and published cases, and exchanged information with support staff, including house (general) physicians. Much of their work consisted of administering, refining, and standardizing reflex tests.

Surgeons assessed whether operation for a tumor was possible, located disease or tissue damage, and removed tumors and repaired lesions. They invented new surgical techniques and instruments and also published cases and technical articles.

Pathologists obtained their own materials, including negotiating permissions for postmortem analyses. They dissected, sectioned, and stained tumors or other tissue and microscopically examined this material.

Physiologists tried to recreate, in animals, the malfunctions of human disease. Their techniques included surgically removing tissue and applying electricity to the exposed cortex to chart nervous pathways and reactions.

As mentioned earlier, the primary focus of my research was on the group based at the National Hospital for the Paralysed and Epileptic, Queen Square. Queen Square was one of the numerous specialty hospitals that developed in mid-nineteenth-century England and was, like many of them, primarily a charity hospital. Although localizationist work was conducted in other countries and sites (especially in Germany, Italy, and the United States), it was developed most clearly and thoroughly, and propagated most widely and succinctly, by this group.

Several important developments changed medical practice during this period: modern brain surgery was developed;[3] antisepsis became accepted and its application standardized; patients were grouped into disease categories in special wards or specialty hospitals instead of being assigned to general wards, facilitating comparative studies; and several methods and techniques for physiological experimentation on animal nervous systems were developed. Researchers culled evidence of localization through a number of techniques. The daily and institutional contexts of this work are analyzed in detail in Chapters 2, 3, and 4. Here I present an overview of the types of evidence they collected and the logic used to justify them.

Autopsies

Although postmortems were not routine in the 1870's, physicians and surgeons had for the most part become familiar with dissection techniques (Lewis 1880). As noted above, Broca's original evidence came from his postmortem examination of the brain of a patient who could not speak. When he found an abnormality in the third frontal convolution of the brain, he declared that this was evidence for the existence of a speech center. This strategy had appeared earlier in physiological work as vitalists searched for control centers in various parts of the brain. For example, Flourens linked breathing with a spot in the lower brain he called the *noeud vital* (vital node). He proved his point by deleting various parts of pigeons' brains and observing the effects on respiration (Olmstead 1944). Investigation into the location of this vital node, as well as into possible alternative centers for respiration, proceeded well into the 1870's (Kellogg 1981).

Experiments

English physiologists eagerly adopted the experimental strategy of deleting parts of the nervous system and observing the consequences. The logic was used both on experimental animals and in observing what Jackson (1873a) called natural experiments of disease in humans, in which parts of the brain were destroyed by pathological processes. The medical journals of the 1870's are filled with detailed examples of postmortem work in which researchers try to link softening, discoloration, or erosion of areas of the brain or nervous system with loss or disturbance of functions. In the early years there were also many reports of failures to find such correlations (see, for example, Gowers 1878; Duncan 1879; Althaus 1880; Ferrier 1881; Hobson 1882; Ross 1882b). These failures provided important ammunition for diffusionist attacks: if correlations occurred only sometimes, then what was the scientific basis for the attribution of specific functions? Researchers also used autopsies to locate nerve pathways from the spinal cord to the brain. They tried to link these paths with localization of functions.

One goal of many of the autopsies at the asylums was to prove that lunatics' brains weighed less than other brains. Though tangential to localization work per se, such work did provide a kind of legitimacy for the autopsies done at places like West Riding. Brain-weight studies were not explicitly localizationist, but they too were part of, and helped legitimate, the search for physical bases of mental disorders (Gould 1981). This allied line of work was often done by localizationist researchers (such as Crichton-Browne 1879, 1880). It continued through the turn of the century.

In Vivo Lesions and Experimental Lesions

The logic of deletion was extended to the location and production of lesions (injuries to tissue). *In vivo* brain lesions can be caused by blows to the head, bullet wounds, or diseases that erode tissue, such as syphilis and tuberculosis. *In vitro* lesions produced on animals can be created by surgical removal of part of the brain, electrical shock that damages tissue in certain areas, or the injection of tissue-destroying substances.

Localizationists used in vivo lesions as examples for localization theory when the lesions interfered with functions (see Gowers 1878; Mills 1879; Shapter 1880; Urquhart 1880; Fraser 1881; Ferrier 1882). For instance, if a patient had a wound on the left side of the head near Broca's speech area and was also speechless, this became confirming evidence for Broca's location of the speech area. Between 1860 and 1910 the journals abounded with cases of patients with partial paralysis or mental impairment after concussions or skull damage in various parts of the head (see Bartholow 1874). These cases were an important source of evidence for localizationists.

Similarly, researchers produced lesions in the laboratory to adduce evidence for the theory. For example, they would surgically open a monkey's skull and remove a part of its brain. If the monkey then developed paralysis on one side of its body, researchers used this as evidence that the deleted brain section had been originally responsible for movement on that side of the body.

The antivivisection movement had an important influence on the in vitro production of lesions (discussed in detail in Chapter 2). Antivivisectionists were opposed to laboratory experiments involving animals and were very powerful in Victorian England (French 1975). Because of their activity, and because of a lack of funding for physiological research, British physicians who wanted to do physiological experiments had either to go abroad for training (to Germany or France), which many of them did, or to serve an apprenticeship with someone already trained. This made the acquisition of skills somewhat idiosyncratic.

There was little agreement between researchers on standard equipment or laboratory procedures. Such diversity frequently characterizes the early stages of research in a field. In brain research, for example, there was no agreement about whether to use faradic or galvanic current; about whether to ablate animal brains with a scalpel or with jets of water; or about how much tissue to take out or how to control surgical complications (see Dodds 1877–78).

Electrical Stimulation

The electrical activity of the brain was first discussed in detail in the report published in 1870 by Fritsch and Hitzig. They applied electrodes to the exposed brain of a monkey and observed movement on a galvanometer. The use of electricity in English medicine was common during this period, so the research methods of Fritsch and Hitzig were easily adapted by British doctors (Schiller 1982). The two scientists' discovery was used to launch a new kind of work in England, applying electricity to parts of the cortex and observing muscle movements. Researchers then claimed that the movements were caused by the part of the brain stimulated.

Electrical work on the brain rapidly became quite detailed. Ferrier applied electrodes to areas as small as one-sixteenth of an inch, and he made functional maps of the brains of various animals based on this precise measurement. (The contemporary form of EEG [electroencephalographic, or brain-wave] technology, which picks up and amplifies the brain's own electrical signals, was not widely used until about 1910 [Brazier 1961].)

Surgery

Surgery on the brain and nervous system existed before the 1860's, but techniques were extremely crude. Even in the 1870's antisepsis had not become universal, and where used, it was often applied unevenly. Patients almost always died of infection after these operations, even if they did not succumb to shock or hemorrhage on the operating table.

The earliest brain surgery was predominantly on skull wounds or abscesses, not on tumors. If someone had a head wound, a surgeon would occasionally be able to remove bone chips or drain off fluid without killing the patient, especially if the dura mater—the membrane surrounding the brain—was not punctured. These early operations were sometimes used to support localization theories. For example, a patient with a concussion on the left side who suffered from right-side paralysis was cured when a piece of bone was removed from the left side of his broken skull. This was seen as evidence for localization of function (MacCormac 1881).

In 1879 the surgeon Victor Horsley performed the first operation using localization theory to locate a tumor in the spine. William Gowers, a neurologist, provided the estimate of where the tumor was located. (Both men were associated with Queen Square for most of their careers.) In 1884 the first brain tumor operation relying on localization theory was performed in London by Rickman Godlee (Bennett and Godlee 1884). Godlee, who was the nephew of renowned surgeon Lord Joseph Lister (Godlee 1917), was in part chosen to do the operation because workers at Queen Square believed that he would adhere to the principles of antisepsis. Hughes Bennett, a physician at Queen Square, provided the neurological information and testing for Godlee's operation. Both of these operations received wide publicity, and medical journals immediately hailed them as turning points. They were also used to justify vivisection experiments (as training for surgeons to work on human brains) and were offered as proof of the clinical usefulness of localization (Spillane 1981).

The relationship between mapping the brain and locating brain tumors is a complex one. Although Godlee's operation was cited as proof that localization theory worked, the cases of patients who entered the National Hospital for the Paralysed and Epileptic with brain tumors were not routinely analyzed to verify localization (National Hospital Records 1870–1901). Rather, exemplary cases in which localization criteria and location of tumor matched were cited in the literature. Even though these were the exception, not the rule, localizationists made claims for their ability to routinely diagnose and locate brain tumors. Such claims, made in a field with almost no other contenders, significantly buttressed the credibility of localization theory.

Pathology and Histology

Pathologists used microscopic evidence in an attempt to demarcate functional areas of the brain. Locating tumors, distinguishing tumor tissue from healthy tissue, and classifying tumors according to their location in brain tissue was an important additional source of evidence for localization of function (Lewis 1878a, 1878b). By the first decade of the twentieth century, new lines of evidence were also developing from histology to support localization. The distribution of different kinds of cells in the brain was correlated with different functions ascribed to those areas (see Campbell 1905). Much of this latter work was refined after 1910.

The Nature of Scientific Theories

Science Is Work

Scientific theories begin with situations: a charity hospital with a mandate, desperate clients having seizures on the doorstep, doctors embedded in a medical profession with a need to appear scientific, antivivisectionists lobbying for an end to those same doctors' experiments. Theories are responses to the contingencies of these situations—courses of action articulated with yet more courses of action.

Nature is a continuous, highly parallel universe of such situations. The theories that scientists form about nature *are* the actions that both meet specific contingencies and frame future solutions.

As George Herbert Mead defined the term "situation," it is an organization of perspectives that "stratifies nature":

> The existence of motion in the passage of events depends not upon what is taking place in an absolute space and time, but upon the relation of a consentient set to a percipient event. Such a relation stratifies nature. These stratifications are not only there in nature but they are the only forms of nature that are there. (1964 [1927]: 315)

Situations are the organization of perspectives, lived experiences. Mead's stance here is radically relativist: "they are the *only* forms of nature that are there." A scientific perspective participates in many such forms.

For most of us, this is an unfamiliar way to think about nature or perception. Perspectives are not ways to "approach" a nature that is already there; instead, the intersection of perspectives stratifies nature and makes it meaningful. Perspectives in this sense are not limited to human beings, though human beings have some unique reflexive capacities. Nor are perspectives a "cognitive" capacity; instead, they refer to practice, experience, and position. In this sense a theory is inseparable from a situation—from its origins, practice, and consequences. That is, scientific theories are work, not disembodied ideas. Or, as Marx and Engels put it:

> We do not set out from what men say, imagine, conceive, nor from men as narrated, thought of, imagined, conceived, in order to arrive at men in the flesh. We set out from real, active men, and on the basis of their real life-process we demonstrate the development of the ideological reflexes and echoes of this life process. . . . Life is not determined by consciousness, but consciousness by life. (Tucker 1978: 154–55)

Many stories have been told about the development of localization theory during the last quarter of the nineteenth century. For some, its appearance is a relapse into phrenology, a revival of the doctrines of Franz Joseph Gall and Johann Spurzheim, never fully weeded out from medical thought. For others, association psychology lent its *geist* to the development of the localizationist movement, and the functional regions of the brain were the logical extension of the philosophy of Alexander Bain (Young 1970; Warren 1921) and other associationists. Association psychology was the idea that thoughts arose from experience and that a complex mental life was formed by thoughts linked in some way (such as similarity, closeness in time, or causally). Some association psychologists postulated a chemical or neurophysiological basis for the links (O'Neil 1985: 48). For most medical historians, however, cerebral localization was simply the discovery of a fact that exists in nature—neither a debate nor a construction, but simply a revelation about anatomy and function.

I began this study with the premise that scientific theories are made, not born, regardless of how I would evaluate their veracity. That is, people do not unearth facts—they assemble, array, propose, and defend them from their situations. One important aspect of this process for scientists is managing the constant uncertainty and complexity that workplaces present (Star 1985a).

Basic questions arise here about the nature of scientific change. There has been much dispute in the history and philosophy of science about the sources of truth for scientific theories. Roughly, these sources fall into two classes: "internalist" explanations, which tend to emphasize logics, ideas, and the progression of events based on the unfolding of ideas; and "externalist" explanations, which account for scientific change on the basis of institutional, political, or other social factors. The debate briefly falls out along these lines: no purely internalist explanation can account for changes in logic that are internally contradictory, nor can a purely externalist one explain the need to reconcile anomalous findings and uncertainties encountered in the course of investigation or explain the nature of contingencies involved in the practice of problem-solving.

Scientific change and stability deeply concern sociologists, historians, and philosophers of science. Thomas Kuhn (1970), for example, has accounted for scientific change via the action of anomalies as catalysts. According to him, anomalies pile up and form the base for a quantum leap into the next paradigm. But in the case of localization, anomalies were used to create a more plastic, thus more durable, theory.

Since the mid-1970's, some sociologists of science have (amid a great deal of controversy) used the concept of "interests" to explain how scientists come to adhere to one theory or another; changes in those interests would then explain why they switch allegiance. Such explanations have been called impoverished because they set up "society" and "science" as somehow distinct, and they fail to explain how society gets into the science. The explanation for scientific change offered in this volume is neither internalist nor externalist; indeed, a major thrust of this and related work in the sociology of science has been to refute the possibility of such a distinction (Gerson 1983a; Collins 1985; Callon, Law, and Rip 1986; Callon 1987; Latour 1987). In order to understand how this works, we first need to analyze the collective nature of scientific action.

Work Is Collective: The Sui Generis Nature of Organizations

Scientific work is collective in nature. The situations that create scientific theories are not single experiments, laboratories, or moments in individual biographies. The stratification of perspectives occurs as a result of numerous interactions and power relationships. The localizationist perspective cannot be reduced to a single fact, a single location, incident, or proponent. As with all scientific theories, its development is a dense interweaving of commitments, heuristics, rationalizations, and truths. As a social fact, it is sui generis and irreducible (see Latour 1987, 1988).

Scientific theories comprise actors in collective enterprise, with a present identifiable existence and an historical dimension. These collective going concerns have personnel, clients, and financial support. They may be well- or ill-organized, old or new, imply a firm mandate for action or none at all (Hughes 1971b: 52–64). To say that a theory *is* collective action is to emphasize my analysis of science as organized practice (Star 1985b).

Thus, to understand truth and scientific theories, we need to understand how collectivities work and how joint action in the course of science is undertaken. To the philosophical sense of truth, then, we add robustness in the sociological sense, and in fact they cannot be separated. Robust findings are collections of actions that, taken singly, may not hold up as valid or reliable, but that *collectively* describe or manipulate the world well enough for a number of purposes. The robustness of a finding or approach is not affected by changing single elements; it is composed of interdependent parts. Robust theories in this sense have historical continuity and enough political allies to guarantee their survival.

This means that a sociological understanding of a scientific theory is not vested in a set of elegant formulas that work together step-by-step to consistently and completely encompass the world. Rather, sociological robustness is found in clumps of workable imperfect techniques, partial sightings, somewhat successful experiments, and local ad hoc alterations to idealized descriptions. The philosopher Arthur F. Bentley gave this kind of robustness the delightful label of "clotted references" (1926).

Sociologically, the emphasis is on the terms "hold up," "collectively," and "well enough" in the preceding paragraphs. As this book shows, each of these terms is problematic for even a small and relatively cohesive group of investigators. Truth, viewed pragmatically, means consequences. In the case of a collective enterprise, it means shared consequences.

Because robustness is a property of collectives, it follows that scientific theories cannot be completely understood from any single vantage point. "No omniscience" is for the sociologist of science the equivalent of the historian's "no Whig history" or "no presentism." It implies a fundamental epistemological democracy, which is the hallmark of sociological analysis. That is, each way of knowing is accorded a certain integrity based on the recognition that different situations create different perspectives (Gerson 1976 calls this a "sovereignty"). This is *not* value-neutrality, but rather the opposite. As a scientist, I can never be exempt from having a perspective; the sociology is in understanding that everyone else does, too. (Whether I agree or disagree with them is a different question.) I will return to this point again below.

Scientific Theories Are Open Systems

The understanding of scientific practice has benefited from fine-grained sociological analysis of the construction of scientific facts—that is, the flow of information and "inscriptions" in the laboratory and in scientific journals (Latour and Woolgar 1979; Law 1985, 1987;

Lynch 1985; Griesemer 1984). Another rich source of analysis comes from computer science. For several years I have been collaborating with a group of researchers at MIT's Artificial Intelligence Laboratory—Carl Hewitt and the Message Passing Semantics Group—on a project to describe problem-solving in the scientific community as a basis for artificial intelligence.

Hewitt has described several characteristics of modern real-world information systems, which he calls "open systems" (1985). His analysis of open system characteristics can be applied to the scientific community (Hewitt and deJong 1984) and to workplaces in general (Hewitt 1985, 1986; Gerson and Star 1986). Hewitt's use of the term "open systems" stands in contrast to information systems based purely on logic or math that assume a closed world, logical consistency, and centralized control. By contrast, he argues that real-world information systems are continuously evolving and decentralized. They require negotiation between distributed parts in order to function, and as a result contain arm's-length relationships between components. The internal consistency of an open system cannot be assured, because its very character is open and evolving.

Information comes into an open system asynchronously: one site may find out about a new piece of information long before another does. The information in an open system is also heterogeneous; that is, different locales have different knowledge sources, viewpoints, and means of accomplishing tasks based on local contingencies.

Scientific workplaces are open systems in Hewitt's sense of the term, and it is a useful term because it reminds us of the decentralized, evolving nature of information. In the scientific workplace, new information is continually being added to the situation in an asynchronous fashion; there is no central "broadcasting" station giving out information simultaneously to scientists. Instead, information is carried piecemeal from site to site, with lags in between of days, months, or years.

Scientific work is decentralized in this way. Thus there is no guarantee that the same information reaches participants at any time, nor that people are working in the same way toward common goals. People's definitions of their situations are fluid and differ sharply by location; the boundaries of a locality are also permeable and fluid. Scientific work is deeply heterogeneous: different viewpoints are constantly being adduced and reconciled. Information from different sources, with different ways of structuring data and different access to data, is continually being added.

Plasticity and Coherence: The Paradox of Open Systems

Within what may sound like near chaos, scientists nevertheless manage to produce robust findings: they are able to create smooth-working procedures and descriptions of nature that hold up well enough in various situations. Their ability to do so was what originally fascinated Hewitt about the scientific community. In the absence of a central authority or standardized protocol, how is robustness achieved? The answer in human systems is complex and twofold: they create theories that are both plastic and coherent, through a collective process of action.

Any scientific theory can thus be described in two ways: the set of actions that meets those local contingencies constantly buffeting investigators, or the set of actions that preserves continuity of information in spite of local contingencies. These are the joint problems of *plasticity* and *coherence*, both of which are required for theories to be robust. Plasticity here means the ability of the theory to adapt to different local circumstances, to meet the heterogeneity of the local requirements of the system. Coherence means the capacity of the theory to incorporate many local circumstances and still retain a recognizable identity.

These problems have remained elusive in the philosophy of science partly because of the failure to understand both the collective and the open systems nature of scientific theories. Scientific truth as actually created is not a point-by-point, elegant, logical creation. Rather, in the words of Richard Levins: "our truth is the intersection of independent lies" (1966). These are not lies in the sense of deliberate mendacity, but rather, necessarily partial truths.

Understanding how scientific theories are formed can be difficult; it is easier to list or name factors that somehow add up to a school of thought or down to a fact. But the dynamics of theories are more than just a hydra-headed list of factors. Each of the actions described in this book contributed in specific ways to a tightly coupled relationship between plasticity and coherence, between practice and theory. The following section discusses some of the dynamics of coherence and plasticity in open problem-solving systems.

The Dynamics of Coherence in Open Systems

Successful scientific theories exhibit a certain amount of inertia, an important basis for coherence. Inertia, in physics, is defined by the statement that a "body in motion stays in motion unless acted upon by some outside force." Successful scientific theories reflect commitments to work practices that are not easily changed. This does not occur as the result of some self-propelling quality of ideas, but rather as the consequence of commitments to training programs, technologies, standards, and vocabularies. Such multiple and overlapping "side bets" are difficult to disentangle or dismantle (Becker 1960).

Furthermore, alliances and conflicts between researchers (Strauss 1978b) make the revision of theories increasingly difficult over time. As more researchers develop a theory's ramifications and adopt them in different kinds of work sites, the theory rapidly becomes complexly rooted. For example, commitments to one size cage entail further commitments to a certain size experimental animal; in turn, the animal's rhythms may dictate a conventional time frame for experiments (see Becker 1982 for a discussion of this phenomenon in the art world).

For scientific change to occur, the payoff for abandoning the theory and its conventions must be higher than the payoff for keeping it. There is an asymmetry involved here, because future research payoff is always uncertain, and what one has in the present, though it may not be perfect, is at least known and tried.

This inertia is implicated in the local versus general applicability of results. Anomalies or difficulties are often perceived as more local than the impact of potential results. This means that there is an asymmetry between perceived problems with a potentially high-payoff solution and perceived advantages for the solution. A problem in achieving clear results is often seen as local to a laboratory; potential payoff for solution from that same laboratory would be seen as having an impact on the entire line of work.

Theories do not develop in single sites, but diffusely and often rapidly. This incurs another important open systems dynamic: momentum, a process that contributes to the plasticity of findings. Momentum in this sense stems not from an intrinsic quality of the ideas at stake, but rather from the social organization of work. There may be many reasons for rapid diffuse growth, including the way in which results from multiple sites are reported by scientists. They are often simplified; the results are reported in a fashion that deletes many of the work contingencies involved in doing the research (Star 1983). That is, when reports of results are made, qualifications and difficulties have often been jettisoned (Latour and Woolgar 1979).

Various types of bandwagons are another source of momentum. They may form around popular notions or techniques (Fujimura 1986, 1988), funneling funding in particular directions or transforming problems into popular terms.

The learning curve holds in science as elsewhere. Thus, by the time difficulties with a theory emerge, inertia has already set in and many conventions have been adopted. There is a honeymoon period in which aspects of a theory or technology may be tried out before flaws in it are taken seriously, but during that period equipment and experimental animals are purchased, clinical training proceeds, and results are published.

Hierarchies of credibility (Becker 1967) form rapidly, and good results reported by prominent investigators at the top of one line of work are picked up and used as valid by researchers in other lines of work. Thus when Nobel prize–winning physicists comment on developments in neurobiology, their word is taken more readily than that of a junior researcher in neurobiology—and the theory endorsed by the physicist gathers momentum across work sites.

Theories do not appear in their entirety in any one site or situation—this is their distributed nature, as discussed above. Although some parts of a theory will often be explicitly developed in one site, a full elaboration of it can only be found on an aggregate level. Theories include tacit local knowledge developed differently in scattered sites. They also reflect widespread assumptions about nature: "that's only natural" or "of course, that's just the way the world is put together" (Garfinkel 1967). All of these conditions preclude comprehensive description from any one point. Temporal factors are also important for incompleteness; theories are constantly in motion, often very rapid motion. Thus, simply keeping up with developments as perspectives are forming is impossible. No one has an "overview" because events are happening too rapidly—one cannot stop the world to describe it in its entirety. Furthermore, updates are made asynchronously to different parts of the scientific community, reflecting the lack of a centralized "update" mechanism or simultaneous broadcast facility.

Pluralism, in the form of different viewpoints, also makes theories incomplete at any one point. All participants in the development of a theory have different (albeit often only slightly different) versions of what is happening. Recall Levins's definition of robustness as "the intersection of independent lies." The aggregate view that emerges from a perspective cannot be robustly represented by any individual viewpoint, since there is never complete agreement about phenomena.

Reification is another important contributor to open systems dynamics. As results are generated and made robust by multiplying commitments (especially institutional, technological, and sentimental), the *origins* of these abstract results in the process of work are forgotten (see Restivo [1983, 1984] for an excellent discussion of this process in the ideologies of "pure" mathematics). The abstractions generated within perspectives are concretized, and the facts are made unproblematic (Dewey 1920). As Mead described these abstractions in his 1917 essay, "Scientific Method and the Individual Thinker": "Their actuality as events is lost in the necessity of their occurrence as expressions of the law" (p. 198).

William C. Wimsatt (1986) discusses another source of reification: the occurrence of what he calls "frozen accidents," unplanned events that happen early in the development of an organism or organization. These events precipitate commitments to ways of working or standard operating procedures that in many cases are awkward or clumsy (Gasser 1984, 1986). Like their analogues in embryological development, these events ramify throughout the system, becoming entwined in all its various aspects. Thus, changing or eradicating their effects at points later in the developmental trajectory is nearly impossible, if only because the expense of doing so is much greater than living with the effects of the frozen accident.

A similar situation has been described by Peter Becker (1983) in his

examination of computer systems used by various firms. Many companies have computer systems that are outdated and unwieldy. If they
could institute a new system from scratch, it would be more efficient.
The old systems, however, grew up gradually, and many standardized
ways of working around them have been built into the company. All
of the company's data and the training of its personnel are invested
in them. To switch to a new system would involve complete retrain-
ing, stopping production, and reentering data. Many of these systems
contain multiple "frozen accidents" in the sense that temporary, un-
official ways of working around a problem became integral parts of
daily routines (Gasser 1986; see also Kling and Scacchi 1982). It would
be too expensive to replace them, since every aspect of the company's
business is somehow and differently involved in the current system.
Although scientists (and the management of the companies Becker
describes) realize that they are living with imperfect, often wrongly
reified results, they cannot afford to change them.

Theories are the end result of many kinds of action, all involving
work: approaches, strategies, technologies, and conventions for investigation. The component parts of a theory become increasingly inseparable as it develops. Again, they become thicker, or "clotted."
Events, observations, and assumptions not logically or practically associated at the beginning of the theory's development come to be
seen by participants as necessarily connected. For example, at the beginning of the localization movement there was little or no necessary
connection between vivisectionist practices and localizationist brain
research. By the end of the period, vivisectionist methods had become inextricably linked with localizationist research. Edward
Sharpey-Schafer (1927) noted that it would have been impossible for
an antivivisectionist approach to be applied to the questions involved.

An Answer to the Puzzle from an
Open Systems Viewpoint

Each of the considerations discussed above appears vividly in the
development of localization theory. I return to the original puzzle:
how and why did localizationists do a theoretical turnabout to maintain internal consistency, without seeming inconsistent to themselves? How did this gradual absorption of anomalies occur? Why did

the discovery of anomalies not undermine, but to all appearances strengthen, the localization model? How did seeming contradictions become transformed into supporting evidence? The answer can only be understood in collective, open systems terms.

The institutional contexts of localizationist research and clinical practice, including medical professionalization and specialization, formed a basis for the rapid technological development and marketing of localization theories. Localizationists were also prominent in medical reform (see Chapter 2). Their careers were linked with the rising and coupled fortunes of localization theory and medical reform.

At the same time, they began their work with and for human subjects who had been abandoned by most of medicine and had little political power (that is, epileptics and other inmates at a "pauper lunatic asylum" and, later, at a localizationist-oriented charity hospital). Their clinical work was thus politically safe during its initial stages. In the asylum and with impoverished populations, they created an area of autonomy and were able to form a strong political basis for their claims of expertise. New experimental programs are routinely conducted on populations with relatively little political power, such as prisoners or mental patients. (See Hornstein and Star, forthcoming, for a discussion of the politics and consequences of such practices for theories of human nature.)

The British antivivisection movement mobilized localizationist physiologists and helped them cohere as a political and professional unit. Unity against antivivisection in the form of the Physiological Society brought them into close alliance with eminent evolutionary biologists. Simultaneously, the different kinds of daily uncertainties in the laboratory, at the bedside, and in the surgical theater were transformed into the unquestioned premises of the map of localized functions of the brain.

The cumulation of evidence from different kinds of research endeavors—such as clinical work and basic research—was another important aspect of the theory's development. Arguments and pools of evidence were combined to support the localization movement; in addition, problems encountered in one realm were often jettisoned into another. Even where findings from one area might not fit the model, findings from another could account for the phenomena. Localizationist audiences were spread over many domains. The theory's bases of power were thus distributed and decentralized: no one domain, experiment, or finding stood well by itself, but the complex combinations of findings and results intersected and became nearly impossible to unravel.

The controversy about localization, far from weakening the theory, actually helped strengthen it in a related fashion. The tactics used by researchers on both sides of the localization debate were many. The debate became so complex, in fact, that it often obscured the significance of anomalous findings, strengthened acceptance of the underlying tenets of localization, and helped make localizationists prominent in the medical press.

The philosophical aspects of the debate and the research were equally clotted. The localizationists' persistent commitment to Cartesian mind/brain parallelism strengthened and was strengthened by the work organization of these researchers. For example, work was often divided into "mind" and "body" domains; the relationship between neurophysiology and psychiatry during this period is a fascinating example of the forging of an important theoretical "necessary connection." Localizationists furthermore became prominent in philosophical debates about the nature of the brain and the mind. They provided new sources of evidence for both psychophysical parallelism and associationism.

Despite the acrimonious debate with diffusionists, and despite unresolved theoretical inconsistencies and clinical failures, the localization movement was so successful that it came to dominate work in medicine, physiology, anatomy, and neuropsychiatry until nearly the present day. Localization research as a going concern formed the basis for the psychosurgery of the 1940's and 1950's; for functional maps of the brain, still in use; for diagnosis and treatment of head wounds and of brain and other spinal and nervous system tumors; and as the working model for many speech and behavioral disorders (see Penfield and Roberts 1959).

The legacy of the localization movement remains with us outside medical and technical domains, as well. Its assumptions underlie the mountain of work on "right-brain/left-brain" thinking that has preoccupied popular psychology since the 1970's. To speak of a speech area in the brain is common. And popular images of brain surgery, brain wave technology, biofeedback, and human evolution often rely on localizationist assumptions.

Although the localizationists won their battle against diffusionism, there are now and have always been holdouts who did not believe in localization of function (Laurence 1977). Much Russian neurophysiology has been diffusionist in nature (Todes 1981). Sporadic and for the most part isolated work of a diffusionist nature has appeared from time to time in the West—for example, the work of Karl Lashley in the 1920's and 1930's (see Lashley 1929).

Cutting-edge work in neurophysiology today appears—like Sherrington's—to incorporate many diffusionist assumptions. The prominent neurophysiologist F. O. Schmitt (1979) has spoken of emergent, distributed cognitive processing. Cybernetic and other cognitive science models appear to have abandoned simpleminded localization of function in favor of complex and diffused models.

Connectionism, a recent popular movement in cognitive science, is a distributed and, as its name implies, connected model of cognitive functioning (Rumelhart et al. 1986). Yet many of these models continue to be influenced in tacit ways by localizationist assumptions, as I discuss in Chapter 7. Furthermore, much of the work done in less rarefied spheres (such as work with learning-disabled children, wounded veterans, stroke victims, incapacitated elders, and those with speech disorders) routinely uses localizationist categories to diagnose and administer to clients.

Were the Localizationists Right?

Everett Hughes would often sensitize his students to the context-dependency and variability of human behavior by reminding them, "It could have been otherwise." That is, though situations may be multiply determined, they are not predestined. Instead, they are a historical coagulation of chance and commitment, what anthropologist Jean Lave has called "mutually structuring events" (1988). The job of social scientists is to understand how these things came together and structured one another—a job made impossible if the phenomena are seen as inevitable.

It might have been otherwise with the localizationists, in several senses. In the history of this project, I first became interested in studying the success of the localization movement when it became clear that it had been variably successful in different countries. Daniel Todes's work on the development of diffusionist perspectives in Russian neurophysiology (1981) provides an important counterpoint to the case of Western Europe. His work was important to me in first suggesting that localization was not a universally held belief—indeed that it had not been adopted across the board by the end of the nineteenth century—and in pointing to several mechanisms influencing the development of Russian brain research (such as the czar's censors, the Revolution, and the role of Sechenov and Pavlov as representatives of materialist science).

In another sense, one arrives at the feeling that it might have been otherwise by going backwards from instances of a published theory to the work of producing it and to the conditions of production. I have divided this book into chapters that present different facets of the production of the localization theory: sets of actions that, viewed in the aggregate, produced a highly robust theory and that, disaggregated, expose both the contingencies and the regularities of scientific work.

But this set of answers will not satisfy the (many) people who still ask, "Were they right? Are you a localizationist?" The answers to these questions are the same, in essence. I am not a neurophysiologist, and at best I am a rank amateur in the world of neurons and reflexes. The *organization* of neurophysiology is my concern here. I am, to paraphrase Jackson's epigraph, neither a localizer nor a diffusionist, but for a different reason.

The question at the heart of many debates in the sociology of science for the past decade is not, "Were the localizationists (or whatever scientific group under scrutiny) right?," but rather, "Under what conditions does studying the work practices of a group of scientists call into question the validity of their results?" I think the answer must be "Only where an ideology of Pure Science or Pure Thought is well developed." Sociologists of science who study laboratory practices, myself among them, are constantly asked whether our findings do not somehow impeach the soundness of the world. If science is made, not found—if it is historically embedded, not timeless—it appears less true. One member of an audience at a conference recently asked me, "But are you saying that science is *only* socially constructed? Doesn't that mean we can believe anything?"

My answer is twofold. The first part concerns the definition of "social." Yes, I believe that science is social and constructed in the sense of being the result of action. But social for me does not mean something apart from practice. Neither is it exclusively human. Rather, it is a *situation* in the way that I have defined it above. The human/natural world is an irreducible continuum; what we can know are the consequences of actions, our own and those of anyone or anything that affects us. The second part of the answer is, of course, we are not free to believe just anything. The idea that we *are* free in this way is what I call the "mere society" argument (Star 1988b). That is, the idea that "if science is social, then we are at liberty to believe anything" rests on a fundamentally flimsy idea of society and its regularities. On the contrary, I think that beliefs and routine practices are some of the most difficult things to conceive, nurture, and change, especially on a wide scale. In this sense I think the localizationists and their allies are a remarkable group, and their situation is well worth our attention.

How to Study Science: Questions of Scale and Method

To what degree did collective organization succeed in creating one view of the brain, and also of human nature, as natural and legitimate? In some ways it is simpler to analyze the "hows" than the "whys" involved in the transformations from the humbler aspects of daily work to localizationist assumptions in medicine, physiology, and science in general. It is easy to think of the commitment to localization as somehow emerging from the spirit of the age in Victorian England: laissez-faire capitalism, materialism, scientism, and new divisions of labor. Such a connection is plausible; intuitively, for example, it is easy to see individualism and free enterprise reflected in a model of the brain that has independent, enterprising parts of its own. However, I feel that a more detailed account is called for, one that includes the material exigencies of daily work and institutional forms. There were important interactions between daily contingencies (such as the clinical management of brain-cancer patients desperate for relief) and larger-scale images, paradigms or pictures of nature that emerged during this period (Daston 1978; Danziger 1982; Richards 1982).

The articulation of large-scale, national changes (such as sweeping economic upheaval, changes in methods of production, wars, national policies, and stratification) with medium- and small-scale organization in science is beginning to be explored. Geoffrey Bowker's research (1984, 1989) on the industrialization of science links changes in work organization and ideas with larger-scale industrial changes in means of production. Elihu Gerson (1983b) has linked problem choice and modeling in evolutionary biology with large-scale funding trends and industrialization at the turn of the century. Bruno Latour's analysis of Louis Pasteur and Pasteurism (1988) ties experimental materials and techniques to empire-building and diplomacy across many sites. Adele Clarke's research (1985) explores the organization of research enterprises across medicine, biology, and agriculture. The work of both Philip Pauly (1984) and Charles Rosenberg (1976) on biology and medicine implies large- to medium-scale influences on problem choice at the institutional and governmental levels.

Although I am concerned with this articulation, much of my work here centers on medium- to small-scale work organization. For example, the epileptics with whom Jackson worked were social castoffs, sent away to charity asylums or hospitals from working- and lower-class families. Doctors often did autopsies on deceased patients from mental asylums for the poor. Several prominent localizationists (including Jackson, Ferrier, James Crichton-Browne, and Bevan Lewis) spent years working in the postmortem rooms and laboratories of these asylums. Ferrier's early experiments were conducted under the auspices of the West Riding Pauper Lunatic Asylum.

This situation had several advantages from the point of view of the physicians. Because impoverished lunatics did not have a high "social value" (Glaser and Strauss 1964) and had often been abandoned by their relatives, effective objections to postmortems were rare. Many of those incarcerated had had syphilis, speech disorders, paralysis, or epilepsy. The asylum setting also provided enough cadavers to make comparative studies possible. For the purposes of linking functional disorders with areas of the brain, the brains of the insane provided an important source of material for examination.

The doctors who administered lunatic asylums in the late nineteenth century had considerable discretion. There were few standard forms of treatment, and there were even small sums of money for research (Viets 1938). In an era when British physiology was almost completely unfunded, even at the university level, the lunatic asylums occasionally provided a place to do basic research. Though resources were not lavish, at least the equipment and subjects for experiments were available. The West Riding Pauper Lunatic Asylum provided such opportunities. It was administered by Crichton-Browne, who later helped found the localizationist journal *Brain*. The other founding editors were Ferrier, Jackson, and John C. Bucknill. Crichton-Browne made it possible for Ferrier and Jackson to do research at West Riding (Ferrier 1873; Jackson, 1873a, 1873b, 1876; Spillane 1981: 389).

I point to this situation (and similar ones involving professionalization, access to resources, and the nature of political alliances) as an indicator of the larger structural variables necessarily involved in making this work possible. The dynamics of power and class, for instance, are clear in the structural position of the patients in the asylums and their witting or unwitting participation as human subjects in experiments. A more thorough analysis of large-scale economic and political contexts of change for scientific theory is beyond the scope of this study, though, I hope, compatible with it and even dependent on it.

Methods and Sources

Unlike contemporary observational studies, historical studies such as this one rely exclusively on documents as data. These documents often omit the details of scientific work processes, or are elliptical about politics, uncertainties, and collectivity. To discover the work processes of localizationists, I examined published work for clues and evidence of simplified results, deletion of descriptions of work processes, and the ways in which different lines of work took for granted or obscured one another's work processes. I also analyzed these processes at several available stages and levels of the work—for example, by examining laboratory notebooks and hospital records, letters, journal articles and their referees' reports, and reports of professional and institutional developments.

During the data collection and analysis, I examined statements made by scientists or historians in terms of the tasks to which they referred. These references were both implicit and explicit. For example, when a scientist claimed that "my experiment proved *x*," I decomposed the phrase into the following sets of tasks:

> a problem was posed;
> monkey bought;
> animal fed and housed;
> skills in surgery and chloroforming acquired;
> an incision made;
> electrodes applied;
> muscle twitches observed;
> twitches coded and written down;
> twitch codes organized and analyzed;
> results noted;
> hypotheses tried out;
> report written;
> report submitted to professional society;
> report refereed and revisions argued about,
>   some included, some ignored;
> report accepted for publication;
> report published.

All of these tasks are compressed into the phrase, "my experiment proved *x*." Moreover, my list is quite short, an incomplete explication of the tasks involved in just one phrase. Scientific literature is full of such phrases. Nevertheless, the above list indicates the way I read such material and the kinds of tasks with which I was concerned. On a larger scale of organization, my lists of tasks included those that occur across many lines of work, such as lobbying for a point of view, ignoring a whole school of thought, and recruiting patients.

Throughout this book I am concerned with the mistakes, as scientists defined them, that they made at work, as well as with their handling of anomalies in the course of constructing arguments and theories. For example, when the experimenter in the above example coded "muscle twitches," how were ambiguous twitches coded? Were they screened out or written down? If a completely unpredictable

muscle twitched—one that could not be explained in terms of the ex-
tant theory—how was that managed? Did the experimenter screen it
out or include it, use it to qualify or expand the theory? Did the ambiguous become a discovery or an exception that could be omitted
from explanations of the phenomenon?

In attending to anomalies and mistakes, I focus especially on their
management—that is, the work associated with defining, locating,
and controlling them. I am not concerned here with evaluating correct or incorrect science, medicine or theories, but rather with helping
to create an analysis of scientific work organization. Scientists themselves make the evaluations. Because they do, and because their evaluations affect the outcome of research, *those* actions are an important
source of sociological data for the study of scientific work.

In this volume I attend to the ways in which scientists merge different types of work to produce a theory. Localizationist physician /
physiologists frequently merged clinical and basic research results to
create a single, unified theory of localization of function in the brain.
Such heterogeneous problem solving and its theoretical and practical
consequences, discussed as triangulation strategies in Chapter 4, is an
important focus of my argument. Such syntheses were common practice for localizationists: results from care of neurological patients,
neurosurgical results, and case histories were combined with animal
experiments and pathological data. In addition to combinations of
clinical and basic evidence, I also found combinations of mechanical
and theoretical work: for example, the application of electrodes to the
brain of a monkey and the development of philosophical theories that
would explain the consequences of the applications. Political and theoretical work combinations were also common, such as in the work
of lobbying for permission to do animal experimentation and in the
development of methodological rationales that included animal experiments.

The combination of disciplinary and other large-scale audiences
with daily, local work considerations is an especially important form
of heterogeneous work. Daily work is the organization of activities
within a single project, and I analyzed this within locales. Disciplinary audiences form a more abstract level of concern, referring to the
ongoing task organization and negotiations of an occupation, discipline, or profession. There was a constant interplay between activities

addressed to daily work and those addressed to the medical and scientific professions at large—for example, getting through a single brain operation with all of its complications and sequelae, and also publishing the results for a general surgical audience or for the discipline of physiology, broadly conceived.

The History of This Analysis

There were several stages in this investigation. After observing scientists at work in a contemporary neurophysiology laboratory (some of the results are reported in Star 1983), I became fascinated with how scientists try to link characteristics of the physical brain with cognition. Scientists at the laboratory were using EEG technology to infer relationships between the brain and behavior. This study left me with the following questions:

1. How do scientists reduce complex data? How do they reconcile the complexity of their findings with constraints and pressures to present simplified results? How are ideas simplified or interpreted in simplified form?

2. How do institutional pressures encourage scientists to choose between styles of theories? Initially, respondents at the lab I observed held a somewhat diffusionist theoretical model of brain function. As government funding for scientific research was slashed, they began to look around for other monies, including clinical funds that relied on application of a highly localized model of the brain. This raised for me the analytic issue of the relationship between funding pressures, career and disciplinary contingencies, and allegiance to a scientific theory.

3. What are the different ways anomalies can be managed in the scientific workplace? I observed respondents managing anomalous data in a variety of ways, such as ignoring outlying cases, rechecking anomalous data, and screening human subjects to minimize uncontrollable artifacts. Anomaly management was an important part of these researchers' work, a possibly critical link between work and published theories.

4. What is the relationship between technology and theory development? I observed researchers doing routine work with various machines, obtaining measurements and recording them, calibrating

the machines, and occasionally substituting one kind of machine for another. Simultaneously, they discussed formal, very abstract theories about the nature of the brain and the mind. The connections between the choice of technology used to collect data and their ultimate interpretation were problematic for these contemporary scientists. How were such connections handled by earlier neuroscientists?

I hoped, by historical comparison, to answer some of these questions. My initial reading made clear the importance of the late nineteenth century as a period of consolidation, and of the Queen Square group as pivotal. As I read more about this period, the complex interaction of institutional, professional, intellectual, and technical concerns also became vivid. I decided to limit the scope of the book to this one historical period and group in order to explore these issues in depth. A brief comparison with modern neurophysiology is presented in the last chapter.

After extensive reading about the 1870–1906 period, and after developing a focus on the group at Queen Square, I went to London to examine hospital and laboratory records. I lived near Queen Square, where the hospital is still in operation. Walking around the wings and wards named after the early localizationists, sitting in the surgical theater, and poring over case records, I believe I was able more vividly to reconstruct the daily lives of those nineteenth-century scientists, doctors, caretakers, and patients.

Each of the chapters that follow explicates one aspect of the development of the localization theory with regard to both plasticity and coherence. Chapter 2 analyzes the institutional and professional contexts of localization work, including professionalization processes and their relationship to the theory. Chapter 3 explores the effects of uncertainty and the transformation of local uncertainties into global certainty. Chapter 4 discusses the integration of clinical and basic evidence in making the localization argument and introduces the notion of triangulation strategies. Chapter 5 describes the debate about localization, the positions of antilocalizationist researchers, and the debate's complexity and multifarious nature. Chapter 6 examines the localizationist approach to the mind/brain relationship, or parallelism, and its base in work organization. Chapter 7 discusses the usefulness of analyzing scientific work organization for understanding how scientists reach robust findings from an open system of collective endeavor. It also discusses the impact of the localization movement on subsequent neurophysiology and brain research, including a brief history of its vicissitudes as, for instance, the underlying basis for psychosurgery.

T W O

The Institutional Contexts
of Localization Research

The fate of localization theory as it emerged at Queen Square was entangled with that of the organizations in which it developed. The theory had an important place in the commitments of several worlds: the profession of medicine and medical specialties, hospitals, and British physiological research. Localization theory became linked with a rising acceptance of "scientific medicine" through a complex series of historical events involving the antivivisection movement, professionalization, and advances in medical technology. The remarkable success of localizationism, and the complex theoretical debate that surrounded it, must be understood in light of these "shared fates" (Bucher 1962).

A theory is both product and production technology: a way of understanding the world as well as the outcome of investigations. Its credibility is linked not only with the credibility of those who hold it, but also with the success or failure of the ventures that house it. That success is only partially dependent on the logical tenets of the theory itself, as much of this book illustrates. Other factors, such as political organization, commitments to methods of work, finances, technological improvements, and practical empirical payoffs, are coupled with the evaluation of the theory. This process of coupling is often forgotten or ignored in discussing the truth of scientific theories. How many people have credited Einstein with inventing the atom bomb but ignored the engineering and defense contingencies surrounding its birth? Similarly, localizationists are credited with discovering cognitive function, whereas the work of surgery, patient care, and medical reform is forgotten. The credibility of localization theory rose, however, as its proponents became successful organizers of medical work in various forms.

That the growth of scientific theories may be linked with the fate of the professions from which they emerge is an interesting and rarely studied phenomenon. According to Rue Bucher and Anselm Strauss (1961), professions grow as emergent, confluent segments, whose parts have different implications at different historical junctures. These segments emerge within professions in various ways: as reform movements, as special interest groups, and as part of the division of labor (Bucher 1962). The shared organization of commitments patterns the flow and change of the emergent profession. These groups with shared commitments form what Strauss (1978a) has called *social worlds*: dynamic groups that are constantly aligning, claiming territory and resources, and merging and splitting (Bucher and Strauss 1961). Rob Kling and Elihu Gerson have made a similar point with respect to scientific and computing social worlds (Gerson 1983a; Kling and Gerson 1977, 1978), and Lawrence Busch's analysis of agricultural science (1982) suggests a similar process. Clarke's work on reproductive science (1987) is a good illustration of the historical process by which segments emerge in a scientific discipline.

But if theories emerge simultaneously with their host professions and organizations as part of social worlds, several important questions are raised. How does timing in the trajectory of the profession in which it develops affect a theory's success? Do theories that develop in well-established organizations have different careers from those developed at the beginning of a professionalization process? What other dimensions are associated when a theory and a profession join fates? How is specialization important here? And finally, because occupations often use research to professionalize, are theories commonly *proved* via the professionalization process itself (Hughes 1966)?

Joan Fujimura's work (1986) on the development of bandwagons and problem formulation in cancer research suggests that the "doability" of a research problem derives in part from its organizational position. The work commitments of the organizations involved in problem formulation and solving must mesh, or align, if work is to proceed. In her example of cancer research, all levels of work must align: materials in the laboratory, a cooperating team, funding from outside sponsors, and an audience in the discipline.

This is not simple agreement—much work proceeds via cooperation in the absence of consensus. It is also not the case that people on the top are seen as right or credible by others; that is true to an extent, but it is mitigated by the presence of multiple angles of vision and perspectives in any nontrivial venture. In science, the answers to who is on top and what exactly constitutes agreement are not generally clear. Theories are locally articulated in different sites as part of a large collective enterprise—in this case, science and medicine—and come to have different importance in different parts of the landscape. To the extent that those different kinds of commitments align and support one another across worlds, the theory is strengthened.

Such was the case with localization theory. It was born at a time when the context of scientific investigation was rapidly changing, and it became rapidly implicated in different ways in different kinds of work organization. The commitments of these parts meshed in various ways to produce doable problems and robust solutions.

In this chapter, I delineate those aspects of change in British medicine and physiology that had the greatest impact on the group at Queen Square. Obviously, a full history of British medicine in the late nineteenth century is beyond the scope of this work. The important point of the chapter is that, by the turn of the century, the group at Queen Square found themselves in an extraordinarily strong position from which to put forth their program of research and treatment.

Hospitals and medical practice in Britain changed greatly during the last quarter of the nineteenth century. The group at Queen Square was in the midst of the changes: as leaders of medical reform, as beneficiaries of changing regulations in medicine and hospitals, and as opponents of the powerful antivivisection movement. In general, the changes in British medicine strongly supported the development of medical entrepreneurship—developing specialist practices and institutions that could form a base for research. For many doctors, including those at Queen Square, specialization was necessary for survival. Scientific research was used to legitimate this specialization, particularly in the context of a highly competitive professional world. Successful specialization depended on referrals and patient demand.

Technical advances in medicine during this period helped with the treatment of some previously incurable illnesses or injuries (or were seen to have the potential to do so). Epileptics, for example, saw the advent of new drugs and diagnostic techniques such as those ad-

vanced at Queen Square. At the same time, medical reform restruc-
tured the profession to equalize the status of surgeons and physicians,
changed licensing regulations, and expanded representation on the
regulating bodies. Those surgeons (either individuals or groups) who
were able to claim technical advances were in a particularly good position to gain influence along with the general rise in status for surgeons.

Medical education changed from an apprenticeship (craft-oriented
occupational training) to programmatic, institutionally affiliated
professional training (Newman 1957). Again, those physicians and
surgeons able to find positions in the new medical educational institutions and to influence educational and training practices were in a
position to become unusually powerful during this period of flux.
And again, the doctors at Queen Square were in an ideal position.
Many of them held teaching positions at hospitals and universities
such as the University of London or King's College; they were active
in forming and leading organizations such as the British Medical Association.

Within these shifting contexts, there were many ill-defined groups.
But localizationist doctor researchers came to form a coherent group,
offering a tightly coupled package of theory, therapy, technology, and
education. Indeed, it was *as a coherent group* that localizationists succeeded with their theory of brain function. On the organizational
level, the coherence consisted in the theory's embeddedness in several
organizational contexts, described below.

The Profession: Chaos and Reform

There is little agreement among social scientists about the meaning
of "profession," but most agree that Western medicine was profes-
sionalized at the end of the nineteenth century.[1] Hughes (1966), citing
T. H. Marshall, defined a profession as encompassing several aspects.
First, it is work organized so that *caveat emptor* cannot be allowed to
prevail. Second, income is sufficient for practitioners to pursue a life
of the mind. Aspiring professionals, he next noted, often use research
to raise their status. Clients, too, play an important part in defining a
profession, although when professions are lodged in complex insti-

tutions, client-practitioner relationships are equally complicated. Finally, the evaluation of mistakes and of good practice is reserved to members of the profession.

English medicine in the 1860–1906 period contains each of these strands, but they are often in conflict with each other. Self-regulation of medicine[2] and claims to scientific precision appeared in conflict with *caveat emptor*, but competition for patients was also fierce and standards were irregular. Poor patients, often without their consent, became experimental subjects for medical researchers (Anderson 1966). There was a hard-fought reform movement within the profession, especially during the 1870's and 1880's, that sought to abolish the medical corporations (that is, the elitist Royal Colleges) and equalize professional membership (McMenemey 1966).

At the same time, doctors were anxious not to be seen as "mere tradesmen." They cultivated "gentlemanly" hobbies and wrote philosophical tracts, emulating the classical traditions of the old medical corporations, models of the classical gentlemanly pursuit of knowledge (Reader 1966; Peterson 1978: 39). Although research, including localization research, was used to legitimate changing medical practice and education (Peterson 1978: 260), it was also attacked by the antivivisection movement, which was dominated by the upper class (French 1975).

In addition, as noted above, medicine and medical education changed from a system based on apprenticeship, private schooling, and private practice to one based on hospital training and practice. This simplified some aspects of medical practice and complicated others. It made specialist doctors, such as those at Queen Square, easier to identify by virtue of their association with specialist hospitals (Peterson 1978: 264–65). It thus facilitated the referral system. But the organization of medical care became more complicated in other ways: the nature of medical welfare in England changed dramatically during this period (public hospitals were created for use by both paying and charity patients, and funds from the growing voluntary hospital movement were used to admit poor patients, often in conjunction with teaching and research needs); there was a rise in public acceptance of hospitals; and professional hospital administration and nursing developed as an occupation (Abel-Smith 1964).

It is clear, then, that no simple narrative of professional changes or directions in English medicine of this period is possible. But several processes important to the development of localization theory emerged from these cross currents. Proponents of the theory were prominent participants in all of the processes of change discussed here: medical reform, specialization, and theoretical and technical entrepreneurship in the form of new training programs, new journals, and new styles of research. By the end of the nineteenth century, they stood at the center of a vastly different medical world. It had become one where practices were more standardized, where entry to the profession was more restricted, and where research and clinical practice were much more tightly coupled. This meant that, as insiders, they had ample opportunity to select patients for research purposes. They were key in helping to shape medical standards and thereby to incorporate their own theories and approaches into curricula and experimental practices.

Many of the initial opponents of localization theory were "old-fashioned" doctors who advocated the traditional system of medicine and medical care. Their opposition seems to have entirely vanished beneath the well-organized localizationists' path. As opponents, they had no clear organization or platform, nor were they themselves researchers. They simply ridiculed the early localizationists as "neo-phrenologists," but this had little discernible effect. Those few opponents who could not be classed with the older generation of English doctors were scattered in various European countries. They also lacked the kind of institutional coherence developed by localizationists.

The group at Queen Square was affected by tranformations in English medicine in many ways. Changes in specialization and the rationalization of training were important for the development of localizationism. It is a precise theory, amenable to rationalization in the enumeration of symptoms and diseases. The shifts in the organization of medical care meant that clinical cases could be fed into a research base in a more systematic fashion, and patients designated as having nervous diseases could come quickly and easily to the attention and care of localizationist researchers.

English medicine underwent many changes after the middle of the

nineteenth century. Until that time, medical training had been idiosyncratic and unspecialized. Coordinated collective action was sporadic, and self-regulation was equally erratic. Licensing was highly local; definitions of good practice varied widely from locale to locale.
Licensing requirements were chaotic and nonuniform. (Even as late
as 1886, there were over nineteen different licensing bodies that could
examine candidates in medicine, surgery, or apothecary [Poynter
1966b].) Requirements for licensing by the medical corporations were
widely varied and often included heavy fees (Roberts 1966).

Licensing and examination inequities were exacerbated by the
rapid proliferation of scientific findings and a simultaneous lack of
standardized curriculum. From the point of view of the examinee, it
became impossible to establish definitively what had to be known for
a given examination (Poynter 1966a). Students had to obtain "insider
information" through tutoring or through sponsorship from the examining bodies. The medical corporations became increasingly exclusive because of this combination of high fees and the need for insider knowledge to pass exams.

In 1858, after years of unsuccessful struggle, Parliament passed the
Medical Reform Act (Little 1932). The act established a General
Medical Council, which created a central registry for doctors and
kept a central, alphabetical list of practitioners. The council was em-
powered to prosecute those practitioners it deemed below standard.
Thus it could define quackery as well as standard medicine (Lyons
1966).

The prosecution and labeling of quacks was an important part of
medicine's attempt to move away from a trade or sales image. As
Mildred Peterson notes, "the essence of quackery was tradesmanship"
(1978: 258), including claims for secret or unique cures, patent medi-
cines, and home-brewed systems of medicine. The 1858 act also abolished regional medical licenses. This further weakened the medical
corporations' monopoly on licensing.

The 1858 act did not go as far as some would have liked. Radical
reformers wanted to abolish the medical corporations altogether and
create one portal into the medical profession. Under this system, all
practitioners would have had to train in medicine, surgery, and phar-
macy. Specialized organizations of physicians, surgeons, and apoth-

ecaries would be merged, thus equalizing the status of all practitioners (Parry and Parry 1976).

From 1832 to 1860, there had been a gradual switch in medical education from an apprenticeship system, or private medical school training, to hospital-based training (Little 1932; Newman 1966). This had several important consequences, but most significant was the access of medical students to a wide variety of cases (and especially to a number of different patients with the same disease). This also marked the beginning of a more uniform professional socialization process. Centralized medical education meant not only occupational skills acquisition, but also a chance for the elites of the medical world to inculcate students with their professional values and loyalties. This was the infrastructure for a self-regulating, autonomous profession.

As training became hospital-based, the curriculum could be standardized. Medical students in the hospitals, unlike apprentices in private practice, could rapidly "walk the wards," surveying large numbers of patients in a single visit. This facilitated a move away from complex assessment of the individual patient and toward quantitative assessments of particular symptom-diagnosis links (Ellis 1966; Reiser 1978). The emphasis on observation and experiences in private practice was replaced by more formal course work, lectures, lab work, and supervised practice. Thus they were able to compare cases and develop more rationalized checklists and diagnostic taxonomies. This formed a basis in practice for modular education. Students could begin to study organ systems and disease types in structured segments and in sequence (Abel-Smith 1964:18).

Outside of the hospital sphere, private practice specialization was also developing. By the 1870's pressure had built within the profession for an exclusively specialist/consulting class of doctors and surgeons. This was consciously modeled on the legal profession, with its division between solicitors and consulting barristers (Abel-Smith 1964:102–12). Such a setup would have taken specialists completely out of competition with general practitioners. Although this system never fully evolved, a significant number of doctors did begin specializing in this fashion. Some standing arrangements between specialists and general practitioners were established (Pound 1967). But, for the most part, specialist practitioners used prestige gained in the specialist hospitals to draw patients from a larger pool.[3]

The Hospitals: Sponsorship and Specialization

The development of specialization was thus important for localizationists. As patient-doctor systems of referral were established, and as specialization itself became legitimate, Queen Square was able to establish a solid position as *the* specialty hospital for nervous diseases, epilepsy, and brain tumors. Localization theory flourished in this context, unchallenged by competitors conducting research based on general practice. Localizationists had an unprecedented number of epileptic, tumor, and other neurological patients for comparison. Their data and expertise in all sorts of nervous disorders were unrivaled in British medicine. Changes in hospital structure also allowed individual researcher/clinicians unprecedented autonomy and authority.

In tandem with the profession of medicine, British hospitals were rapidly changing during the last half of the nineteenth century. The various types of hospitals and their legal and bureaucratic conditions were Byzantine in organization, but a number of reforms established or changed the nature of free medical care for the poor, including the establishment and abolition of workhouses and asylums. Because Queen Square was a specialist voluntary hospital, most of this discussion will emphasize changes in this type of organizational structure. It should be borne in mind, however, that all hospitals were undergoing organizational turmoil at the time. For instance, financial grounds for admissions were often unclear. The definition of pauper or charity case varied from beggars to servants or tradespeople unable to finance medical care. Other screening criteria were equally vague. It was unclear whom to screen or admit under the definitions of incurable or acutely ill. There was uncertainty about who had what kind of disease and what kind of specialist had jurisdiction where. And finally, after general funds had been raised to give to the hospitals, it was unclear which funds should go to which hospital for what purpose.

Hospitals in general became increasingly oriented toward teaching and research during this period. Hospital staffs became jointly responsible—with medical schools—for medical education. A standardized curriculum made both education and care more comparable across training sites. Students were allowed to meet curricular requirements by taking courses at different hospital schools (Peterson 1978: 60–77).

As hospitals became the locus of much more medical care during the 1840's and 1850's, an organizational bottleneck rapidly developed. The consulting physicians from Oxford or Cambridge controlled the medical corporations, medical education, and patient fees. There was a sharp division between staff doctors and the consultants at the top of the hierarchy. Hospitals kept staff doctors with junior appointments on low salaries and forbade them from developing private practices. But even these less advantageous staff positions could be obtained only by payment to a consulting doctor.

Jose Parry and Noel Parry (1976: 137) point out that, although hospital appointments for the consulting physicians were not directly remunerative, they conferred a great deal of prestige. Through the system of payments and appointments, the consultants controlled medical students and junior staff. They could use the hospital network as a way to develop a lucrative private practice from patient referrals.

By 1860 there were many frustrated junior staff in the hospitals. House staff were in fact doing much of the patient care but getting little in the way of money, prestige, or hope for advancement. Brian Abel-Smith (1964: 21) estimated that in 1860 there were 15,000 medical practitioners in England. Of these, 1,200 worked in voluntary hospitals, and only 579 were physicians and surgeons in charge of inpatients. The rest were house staff and assistants. In the large teaching hospitals, general practitioners who had taken charge of much general patient care were gradually squeezed out. They were replaced by junior staff who fed cases up to senior consultants.

One way out of the frustrating junior position was to set up an independent specialty hospital (Newman 1966). Between 1860 and 1870, some 30 specialist hospitals were founded, the majority of them by doctors (Evans and Howard 1936: 153). Sixteen of these were in London. The specialties ranged from cancer, nervous diseases and epilepsy, fever, and maternity to bladder stones, electrotherapy, and homeopathy. There was even a special hospital for ulcerated legs.

Given the hierarchical "funnel" structure of hospital organization in the general hospitals, it was difficult for most practitioners to conduct research using wide-ranging comparisons. But specialist hospitals created further opportunities for medical researchers to isolate disease types and thus amass material for comparative cases. Specialist hospitals formed much of the organizational base for specialist clinical research.

The specialty hospitals, not surprisingly, drew criticism from those at the top of the hierarchy. But they were defended by the younger specialists attempting to break away from the bottlenecks created by general consultant control. An 1863 letter from the founder of the London Galvanic Hospital, in response to such criticism, states that this specialist hospital was not established until "after I had failed in my endeavour to become connected with my 'alma mater,' St. Bartholomew's." He was prepared to relinquish the specialty hospital "upon being placed in an established London Hospital, in an honourable and independent position" (*The Lancet* 1 [1863]: 219, cited in Abel-Smith 1964: 29).

The National Hospital for the Paralysed and Epileptic at Queen Square, though not founded by doctors,[4] immediately came to serve the multiple purposes of other specialist hospitals. Its structure allowed career advancement and monetary gain, escape from the consultant-dominated general hospitals, and a chance to conduct clinical research comparing patients with different nervous diseases.

Ironically, the organizational structure of the specialist hospitals, though created in rebellion against the bottlenecked hierarchy of the general voluntary hospitals, often replicated that hierarchy. Consulting physicians and surgeons at Queen Square, for instance, were not paid for their services to patients there. Instead, they developed private practices and held teaching appointments. Their practices were advertised via the publicity garnered from the research and clinical activities at Queen Square. Consulting physicians such as Ferrier and Jackson culled cases for publication, met wealthy hospital sponsors, and exhibited their patients to classes at local medical schools, especially University College (Holmes 1954). Salaried house staff did most of the caretaking, and physicians Jackson, Ferrier, and Gowers visited patients only once or twice a week.

In general, voluntary hospitals were charitable hospitals intended to serve the working-class servants and tradespeople (not paupers). Patients were admitted with a letter of backing from a subscriber, who promised to pay for their care. Often, patients were servants of wealthy sponsors. An additional source of general patient funds came from large-scale fund-raising drives that collected money for hospitals.

The number of voluntary hospitals rose rapidly in the last half of the century. There were 11,000 beds in voluntary hospitals in 1861; by 1891 the number had doubled, and in general they were large organizations (Pinker 1966). By contrast, the specialist hospitals were relatively few and quite small in size, with an average of 36–89 beds apiece. Queen Square had about 60 beds during this entire period. Thus the "sieve" for specialist patients was fairly fine. This reflected several things: the crude diagnostic techniques used by most physicians for many of the illnesses, such as brain tumors and stroke; the control exercised by the larger hospitals; and the size and funding constraints of the smaller specialty hospitals.

An important influence on the nature of hospital care in this period was the emergence of professional nursing. Nurses with the new Nightingale-type training, who were for the most part upper-class, educated women, began to take over much of the care formerly done by uneducated porters, nurses, or surgeons (Dainton 1961: 125–26). These women formed alliances with the upper-class hospital governors and patrons. They thereby established nursing empires within the hospitals, often displacing existing staff. Because the hospital governors were not inclined, for the most part, to involve themselves in clinical decisions, the nurses were free to take over much of the daily care of patients. This in turn freed doctors to diagnose, perform experimental procedures and establish specialist/consulting practices (Abel-Smith 1964: 68).

The Shift to Acute Care and Patients as "Experimental Material"

Localizationist researchers had conducted a series of experiments at the West Riding Pauper Lunatic Asylum during the 1860's and early 1870's (West Riding Pauper Lunatic Asylum 1871–74; Viets 1938). This institution was admininstered by Crichton-Browne, later a founder of the localizationist journal *Brain*. As mentioned earlier, Ferrier's early animal experiments were conducted there. West Riding was also the locus for many reports of postmortem observations of inmates' brains and speculations about the physiology of mental illness (including the cranial capacity of the mentally ill). Many of Jackson's early theories about localization and epilepsy were inaugurated there. From West Riding, after the early 1870's, the center of British localizationism moved to Queen Square.

The original founders of Queen Square had wanted the hospital to be a place for the chronically ill, incurable epileptics, and paralytics. They were especially interested in patients who had no recourse but the workhouses and pauper asylums. However, a doctor who took part in the early planning stages insisted that the hospital allow only *acutely* ill patients. He was able successfully to overturn the founders' wishes (Holmes 1954). This move, in 1860, reflected the widespread movement on the part of voluntary hospitals to deal exclusively with acutely ill patients. There were two reasons for this: one rooted in the research needs of doctor/scientists, the other based on financial and political pressures.

First, the shift to acute care and the development of situations where doctors could do more experimentation was advantageous for the development of theories like localization of function. The rising importance of comparative cases in medical research reflected changed emphasis throughout the profession on clearly defined classes of disease supported by empirical, scientific observations. The more rapid turnover of patients allowed researchers to develop fine-grained taxonomies of localizationist disease by comparing across patients. Without the burden of long-term care for chronically ill patients, localizationist doctors could process and publish cases at a much more rapid rate. They could also select the most interesting and dramatic cases to illustrate their theoretical points.

Second, since the voluntary hospitals were dependent on the charity of rich sponsors for patients, it was important to assure their sponsors that they were handling the largest possible number of patients. There was a distinct advantage, when appealing for funds, in treating acute rather than chronic cases. "The more acute the cases admitted, the greater were the number of inpatients that could be treated in a given number of beds during the year. Such statistics were valuable for appeal purposes" (Abel-Smith 1964: 39).

But doctors did not simply want larger numbers of patients. They wanted control of the hospitals. This became apparent when subscribers attempted to use the hospitals not only as pet charities, but also as private infirmaries. When they attempted to have their personal servants (or tradespeople of their acquaintance) admitted to Queen Square, fights about diagnosis and control of admissions ensued (Abel-Smith 1964: 37).

Throughout the 1860's and 1870's, doctors gained control of hospital admissions. They employed several strategies, such as creating a number of limited-purpose emergency rooms. There, a small number of acutely ill patients could be directly admitted by doctors. This provision bypassed the system of sponsorship and sponsoring letters. As time went on, it formed the organizational basis for untrammeled physician control of the hospital. Patients thus admitted were paid for out of general, uncommitted hospital funds (Peterson 1978: 175). Doctors also banded together and gained control of administrative procedures and meetings. They began to use their scientific reputations, acquired at the specialty hospitals, to barter for more clinical discretion.

Institutional care for the chronically ill poor had been relegated to the poor workhouses until 1866; sick indigents were not admitted to voluntary hospitals. Between 1870 and 1900, there was a gradual conversion of pauper workhouses and infirmaries to general hospitals (Abel-Smith 1964: 127–30). After the late 1880's, researchers began to learn more about infectious diseases in the poor population, hitherto neglected because of these administrative arrangements.

As is characteristic of much medical history and sociology, the story of patients' experience and participation in their care or diagnosis is missing from reports I read of nineteenth-century British neurology and surgery (see discussion of this in Strauss 1979). As I read accounts of brain operations and treatments for epilepsy, and as I looked at photographs of brain tumor patients in the Queen Square casebook, I tried to imagine the patients' experience, daily lives, and participation in their care. Although descriptive material is unavailable, some information can be inferred from the records and the organizational arrangements they portray.

For example, specialists convinced both patients and sponsors, as well as general practitioners, that certain diseases or symptoms could best be managed by specialist hospitals. Patients with a broad range of problems sought admission to Queen Square. They learned that an inability to speak, severe headache, and tremors could indicate nervous system dysfunctions. In addition to obvious symptoms, like epileptic seizures and paralysis, these more subtle symptoms were analyzed and treated at Queen Square.

More important, patients with nervous diseases learned to describe their symptoms in ways that would fit evolving medical taxonomies. Hospital records from the 1860's show only simple, narrative descriptions of epileptic fits in initial interviews with patients. These would include patients' estimates of the conditions that predisposed them to seizures or paralysis. Riding in an open carriage and getting caught in a draft, for example, were two possibilities hypothesized by patients as recorded in the National Hospital files. By the 1880's, doctors had developed methods for channeling and standardizing patient descriptions. They created standardized forms upon which to record seizures, vital signs, and reflex responses. Because many of the patients suffered from frequent seizures, they could not be monitored by hospital personnel. In learning self-monitoring they also acquired a more sophisticated understanding of the basic precepts of localization with regard to epilepsy. Patients learned to report about seizures in detail, with attention to localization-significant signs. This included tracking the progression of twitches over the various muscle groups, locating the muscular contractions, and trying to time the intervals between seizures.

Some patients carried this faith fairly far. Horsley (1904) recorded an instance in his casebook where the mother of an epileptic boy requested a brain operation for his condition. From Horsley's notes, it is clear that she desperately hoped the surgeon could provide a cure for the illness. We know that patient demands affect doctors' practices, so—bearing in mind how much competition there was for patients during this time—we know that patients' beliefs must not have been trivial to the success of localizationist practice.

As noted above, patients at the voluntary hospitals were usually charity cases. In later years, a few paying patients were accepted at some of these institutions. At Queen Square, a paying-patients ward was developed in 1875, but it was almost never fully utilized (Holmes 1954: 18). Abel-Smith (1964: 18) has suggested that a tacit bargain was struck between specialist doctors and charity patients: their free care was predicated on cooperation in experimental procedures. At Queen Square, this cooperation was certainly also predicated on desperation: there was simply nowhere else to go, other than custodial-care asylums, for the poor or working class with severe epilepsy.

Because seizures are a common symptom of brain tumors, the presence of seizures helped direct tumor patients to Queen Square. (Recall the patient who arrived by train at Queen Square with the label "Fits Hospital" literally attached to his coat.) Although effective seizure-controlling drugs were developed in the 1840's, their use did not become widespread until the 1860's (Temkin 1945). But by the turn of the century, the staff at Queen Square was dispensing some two and a half *tons* of potassium bromide, an antiepileptic medication, to its patients every year (Rawlings 1913).

British Physiology: Weak Research Programs and a Common Enemy

From 1840 to 1870 British physiology languished, especially by comparison with developments in France and Germany (Geison 1972, 1978; Rothschuh 1973: 305–6). The lack of developments and discoveries, and the slow growth of British laboratories and professional positions, can be linked with a number of institutional factors. England lacked the highly organized, competitive, and state-supported university systems such as those developed by France and Germany. Instead, organizations were isolated, and the state was not particularly interested in supporting basic science. Science was seen as a hobby for gentlemen, and that model persisted through about 1870.

One consequence of this weak institutional base was that there was virtually no professional physiology outside of medical schools before 1870. In that year, Michael Foster was appointed praelector of physiology at Cambridge University. John Burdon-Sanderson became professor of practical physiology and histology at University College, London, with Edward Schafer (who later changed his name to Sharpey-Schafer) as his assistant (French 1975: 42).

Even after 1870, however, institutional support for physiology was slow to develop. Before that year, English medical physiology had been strongly oriented toward anatomical and structural approaches. That is, anatomical dissection formed the basis for analysis of function. During the early part of the century, this was not much at odds with physiology as practiced in other countries. But the tradition continued in England long after it had been transformed in France and Germany by such investigators as Claude Bernard and Carl Ludwig. So, although jobs for physiologists began to open up after 1870 in English medical schools, they were still tied to anatomical methods, which often excluded good experimental facilities (Geison 1978).

For those who wished to pursue medical/physiological research on a full-time basis, then, the situation was limited. Richard French contrasts the situation of medical researchers with the medical profession as a whole: as a group, researchers lacked autonomy and found an ill-developed institutional base for experimental medicine. "Insofar as they considered themselves scientists rather than healers, their political strength as an occupational group or nascent profession was negligible" (1975: 151).

Whereas in Germany and France physiologists had begun to base their science on chemistry and physics, and to make alliances and design laboratories on this basis, such was not the case in England. The fate of English physiology, then—certainly through the 1870's and, in my opinion, through the turn of the century—was entirely dependent on the fate of medicine. As Gerald Geison says, "In so pragmatic a setting as Victorian England, it should not surprise us that physiology could expand and ultimately secure its independence from anatomy only by exploiting its traditional role in medical education" (1978: 153). This was true both in the treatment-oriented nature of problems selected and in the kinds of equipment and laboratories that were made available. And nowhere was this more true than in the study of localization of brain function.

Localizationist investigators pursuing physiological questions entered an institutional context that was theoretically disorganized, scattered throughout the various medical schools and hospitals, and biased toward investigations of anatomy and function with direct practical, clinical payoff. Equipment for physiochemical or metabolic experiments was scarce, as was support from physicists and chemists. But disorganization and a lack of centralized funding was not altogether a bad thing from the point of view of localizationist researchers. Insofar as researchers remained within the constraints of medical work, they could expect neutrality or mild support from colleagues not directly involved in debates about localizationism. They worked in a field relatively untrammeled by entrenched research interests.

The single most important opponent of localization research was thus not established physiology per se. Instead, it was the antivivisection movement, which condemned all research on live animals. Ironically, however, antivivisection succeeded in uniting English physiologists rather than eradicating them. The Physiological Society was formed by British scientists in 1876 in direct response to antivivisectionists' attacks on investigations. Its first purpose was to protect the interests of experimentalists. In the original society were Burdon-Sanderson, Sharpey-Schafer, Foster, Ferrier, and Jackson—a group comprising all of the professional nonmedical physiologists in England and two of the most prominent localizationists (Sharpey-Schafer 1927).

The Cruelty to Animals Act of 1876, originated and supported by the antivivisectionists, stipulated that anyone performing experiments on living vertebrates must submit an application to the Home Office and be licensed by it. This application had to be endorsed by one of the medical corporations or the Royal Society, as well as by a professor of medicine or medical science. Moreover, the experiments had to be performed at a place registered with the Home Office; these places were subject to unannounced inspection at any time (French 1975: 143). Thus, physiological investigators employing vivisectional techniques were legally, as well as politically, bound by the approval of the medical profession after 1876.

The act of 1876 helped vivisectionists to form alliances with researchers from other sciences, particularly from evolutionary theory. This is reflected in the roster of charter members of the Physiological Society, which included many prominent evolutionary biologists. Among the biologists who supported vivisectionist research were Darwin, Huxley, George Rolleston, and Joseph Hooker, then president of the Royal Society (French 1975: 152). Ferrier was elected a Fellow of the Royal Society in 1876, at the height of the controversy.

In 1881 the International Medical Congress was held in London. This prestigious convention was widely publicized, and the Physiological Society took an active part in the program. At that congress Ferrier confronted the German antilocalizationist Friedrich Goltz, and, in a heated debate, he was said to have definitively defeated Goltz

(MacCormac 1881; Thorwald 1959). Another important outcome of that debate concerned not localization per se, but rather the position of research with regard to vivisection. Many of the statements read to the Physiology Section (including Foster's opening address) focused on the importance of vivisection for physiological research. They deplored the "antiscientific backwardness" of the antivivisection movement. The claims of clinical and scientific advancement made at the congress were sweeping and well publicized.

After the congress and the Ferrier-Goltz debate, the Victoria Street Society (an antivivisectionist group) decided to prosecute Ferrier under the 1876 act. It accused him of having performed surgery without a license on the monkeys he had used to demonstrate his points about localization at the international congress. Ferrier was arrested and put on trial, where it was revealed that Gerald Yeo, Ferrier's associate, had performed the actual surgery. Yeo was licensed by the Home Office to conduct such experiments, and Ferrier was accordingly acquitted. Meanwhile, his trial had attracted the attention of the medical profession and the popular press. The professional associations were outraged by his arrest, and the trial became a key event in developing professional solidarity against antivivisectionists. (See, for example, the discussion in the notes of the Medical Society of University College, in which the association voted to support Ferrier [University College Hospital, "Minutes of the Medical Society," vol. 8, December 7, 1881], and the editorial in the *British Medical Journal* [1881].) The British Medical Association underwrote the costs of Ferrier's defense, and its lawyer represented him in court (French 1975: 202).

At least in part because of the timing of the trial, and because it had been occasioned by the International Medical Congress, the issues of scientific method, vivisection, medical professionalism, and localization theory became inextricably intertwined in the minds of the profession and the public. An even firmer alliance against the common enemy of antivivisection was thus forged between the Physiological Society and the medical profession (French 1975: 203). Localization research was central in this alliance, both because it was an important research topic for the principal actors in the events of 1881 and because it had become a touchstone representing sciences to the public. Thus professional autonomy for medicine, including the freedom to conduct and evaluate research, were symbolically intertwined with both localization theory and vivisectionist physiological research.

The publicity received in the antivivisection battle by Ferrier (and later by Horsley) was a double-edged sword, damaging antivivisectionist support for the hospital but bringing scientific notoriety. Many of the governors of Queen Square were antivivisectionists and did not approve of the experimental work done by its staff. Burford Rawlings, a long-time administrator at Queen Square, said that the hospital lost "thousands of pounds" in donations because of the publicity given to Ferrier's experiments (1913). Perhaps the hospital governors were assuaged by the potential success of brain surgery and the clinical potential of other localizationist-oriented treatments. Brain surgery, in particular, purported to use principles directly derived from Ferrier's experiments to locate brain tumors. After 1884 this became an important source of prestige and international acclaim for Queen Square.

The publicity afforded Ferrier by the trial did wonders for his private practice, which flourished. Because of the consulting structure of medical practice at Queen Square, this was an important turning point in his career and finances. The conduct of his physiological experimentation at that time was dependent on his personal financial resources; experiments were all privately funded and essentially out-of-pocket, except for a small grant from the Royal Society in the early 1870's.

The events of the International Medical Congress and the subsequent trial also revealed an extensive collegial network, based only partly on the fight against antivivisection. Some of the connections involved publications: for example, Rolleston was one of the referees of the Royal Society who accepted Ferrier's first paper for publication by the society (see Rolleston 1874). Burdon-Sanderson hired Ferrier to come to London to do physiological experiments after his early work at the West Riding asylum.

Other links were through theoretical allegiances. Horsley, the first brain surgeon at Queen Square, was Sharpey-Schafer's student and collaborator at University College. Charlton Bastian, a physician at Queen Square, was Spencer's literary trustee and a friend and co-worker of Darwin, Huxley, and Russell Wallace (Holmes 1954: 39). Jackson, also a physician at Queen Square and a leading localization theorist, was heavily and explicitly indebted to Spencer for his theo-retical assumptions (see, for example, Jackson 1932a). Moreover, Jack-son was in a position to influence medical theories through his con-nection with *The Lancet*; he had a great deal of control over what was published there. (According to his biographer, James Taylor, he would often write a short fragment and get the *Lancet* staff to include it even after they had finished the pasteup for an issue [Jackson 1925: 19].)

In sum, British physiology emerged from a tight network of re-searchers and friends who were ideologically allied on many issues. Localizationists were at the heart of this network and were thus able to mobilize its resources for both scientific purposes and personal credibility. Instead of bucking an established tradition, they were in-novators in a relatively clear field, thus augmenting the effectiveness of the interconnections.

Technical Advances in Medicine and the Rise of Neurosurgery

The first successful removal of a brain tumor based on localization theory was performed in 1884 by the surgeon Rickman Godlee with neurological localization diagnosis by the Queen Square physician Hughes Bennett (Bennett and Godlee 1884). The patient survived the operation itself but died 28 days later (Spillane 1981: 398). Still, this was considered a breakthrough. Before that time, doctors had viewed brain surgery as impossible except for the repair of concussion or ab-scess that did not penetrate the brain tissue itself (Cushing 1905). Fol-lowing the 1884 operation, localizationists and surgeons collaborated on a number of operations (Horrax 1952; Sachs 1952). These were closely followed and publicized by the medical press. By 1900, Queen Square was performing 100 operations a year for brain and other ner-vous system tumors (Critchley 1949; Blackwood 1961).

Many medical historians reconstruct a straight line between Fer-rier's animal experiments of the 1870's and the location and successful removal of a tumor from the brain. This is nonsense. Successful brain surgery, including the removal of brain tumors, evolved from a long series of technical improvements in surgery of the nervous system and skull, including better control of bleeding, the invention of new tools and surgical techniques, and, as a crucial step, the discovery and acceptance of antisepsis.

As noted above, Godlee was selected by localizationist physicians to perform the first brain tumor operation because it was known that he would use antiseptic techniques (Thorwald 1959; Spillane 1981). Ferrier and Jackson were present at the operation. Bennett and Godlee's report of the operation in *The Lancet* was widely publicized, in England and internationally, especially by the doctors at Queen Square. The operation heralded a new era in intracranial surgery; it cemented a merger of work interests between neurology and surgery, an intersection based on localizationist theories of nerve and brain function (Cushing 1905, 1910, 1913).

Even after surgical techniques were developed, there was still no one-to-one correlation between symptoms thought to point to a tumor or abscess in a certain area ("localizing signs") and the actual location of such a tumor. But surgeons and neurologists *claimed* that brain tumor operations proved the theory of localization of function. These claims were highly persuasive and benefited both surgery and neurology.

The state of affairs in 1884 was ripe for the merger of interests between the two specialties; what the one had, the other lacked, and vice versa. On the one hand, surgeons had developed increasingly sophisticated skills for nervous system and cranial operations (Rogers 1930); Sir William MacCormac, in Scotland, had performed a number of successful trephining and brain abscess operations using antiseptic surgery (MacCormac 1880). But surgeons lacked physiological theories, pathological training, or even functional explanations that could be used to help make their techniques clinically effective and thus help equalize their clinical status. Neurologists, on the other hand, had many theories but a poverty of clinical techniques. They relied heavily on iodides and electrotherapy for treatment; neither were often successful (Cushing 1910).

Before the mid-1880's, patients with brain tumors or brain abscesses seeking help from neurologists or surgeons faced incorrect diagnosis and, sometimes, incarceration in lunatic asylums; death was almost certain if they risked a brain tumor removal (Cushing 1905). After the 1884 operation, yet more surgical techniques were invented to improve patient mortality rates for brain tumor and abscess operations (Rogers 1930). Horsley, for example, who was appointed to Queen Square in 1886, developed a new bone wax that helped stop bleeding from the skull (Paget 1919). He was also an avid supporter of antiseptic techniques and became well known for his work with Pasteur on the famous rabies research. Surgeons invented topographical measurement methods that made it possible to locate specific areas of the brain underneath the skull and to drill the smallest possible holes in the skull for precise surgery. "Listerism," or antisepsis, gradually became standard operating procedure by the turn of the century (MacCormac 1880), and surgeons' assistants became more expert in the administration of chloroform, thus decreasing the number of accidental deaths arising from anesthetic overdose.

The surgery/neurology intersection, then, became a powerful base for localizationism. The application of localization theory to brain tumor removal was claimed as a clinical justification for vivisection techniques, and the "cure" of a hitherto mysterious and hopeless set of diseases was claimed as a potential, if not actual, victory for localization theory.

Summary: Theories and Work Contexts

From the description of the institutional and professional contexts of localization work, it is clear that localization theory was embedded in the structure of work commitments of several different, though intertwined, enterprises. Localizationists had multiple organizational supports and circumstances for their theory. In concert, these created an extremely sturdy base for the success of the theory. It was "fed" by specialization, by the switch to acute care, by the state of British physiology, and by the professionalization of medicine. None of these factors was alone sufficient to account for its success, but together they were a formidable organizational package.

It is important to contrast the well-organized, tightly knit group of localizationists in the late nineteenth century with the organizational base of the diffusionists in England during this period. Diffusionist criticism was more in the character of "voices from abroad" than of well-organized opposition. These voices were widely scattered and had no support in England comparable to that of the localizationists. Antilocalizationists were not even organized in their criticism of localizationism: I could find no evidence of diffusionist research or criticism permanently based in England after 1870. The three major critics of the group at Queen Square were based in different countries: Goltz in Germany, Mario Panizza in Italy, and Brown-Séquard primarily in France and the United States. Although these critics cited one another's work, they did not collaborate or form professional organizations (see discussion in Chapter 5). And, though they were all eminent, their points of view came to have decreasing plausibility over the period studied here. In part, their experience was the inverse mirror image of that of the localizationists: the diffusionists formed no professional alliances in England; the theories they espoused were not particularly entangled with other successful ventures; they did not "enroll allies" in the same way the proponents of localization did (Latour 1988); and they did not have organizational authority over their opponents.

In sum, then, the professional and institutional contexts within which localizationist researchers worked formed the basis for the success of localization theory. This is not a question of interests nor of perceiving a kind of backdrop to theory development. That is, one cannot identify "external factors" that merely "influenced" the development and success of this theory. Instead, its growth and success were a seamless web of successive events developmentally superimposed on one another. The commitments made by researchers at one juncture, such as the commitment to vivisection, came to limit or create options at a later time, such as the commitment to clinical justification of results. The nature of evidence was thus progressively determined by collective experience.

The organizational and professional commitments described in this chapter are further elaborated and informed by the daily work practices and conflicts of researchers. These include the hands-on aspects of hammering out theoretical details and articulation of the varieties of work that go into a theory-making concern. Daily work and its structure and uncertainties are discussed in the following two chapters.

THREE

Uncertainty and Scientific Work

A classification is not a bare transcript or duplicate of some finished
and done-for arrangement preexisting in nature. It is rather a rep-
ertory of weapons for attack upon the future and the unknown.
—John Dewey (1920: 154)

The following two chapters detail the strategies by
which localizationist researchers created certainty and closure for
their theory. They speak to an important aspect of scientific knowledge: its distributed nature. At no one point in time or space can a
piece of scientific evidence, or even the work or beliefs of one scientist, be said to represent a theory in its entirety. Instead, theories are
actions distributed over multiple sites and long periods of time. No
central authority evolves, adjudicates, or disseminates theories.

This has some important implications for our understanding of
the growth of scientific knowledge. First, the bits and pieces collectively assembled to produce scientific knowledge are heterogeneous
(Law 1987; Star 1988a). That is, because there is no central authority
or distribution system, each locality and each work site develops its
own approaches and its own knowledge about phenomena. When
these are combined, it is as heterogeneous parts; the whole is an ever-
evolving, decentralized system, always incomplete at any one point.

Localization theory became simultaneously embedded in several
different kinds of work and professional contexts, as discussed in the
previous chapter. The cumulative effect of such embeddedness was
the theory's rapid ascendance from a dubious hypothesis to a fact. In
this chapter, we turn to a more fine-grained analysis of the theory's
development. The daily work of medicine and research, its contingencies and structure, is of equal importance with larger-scale orga-

nizational structure in a theory's development. Science grows from the immediacy of a scientific investigator's concerns at the bedside or in the laboratory to broader-based, enduring, and cross-organizational phenomena. I am concerned here with analyzing the transformation of such local contingencies in creating generalized facts. At the heart of this transformation is the management and resolution of uncertainty.

The commitment of localizationists to a model of brain function that would locate behaviors in a physical substrate began in a time of professional and scientific upheaval, as the previous chapter illustrated. In medicine, physiology, and other areas of science that touched on the "mind" or "soul," there were heated debates about human nature, the limits of science, and the notion of "progress." New technologies abounded and made possible whole ranges of new experiments. The stakes for demonstrating a scientific, physical basis for the mind were extraordinarily high (Daston 1978; Danziger 1982; Richards 1982). To do so would have been a major advance for scientific materialism, evolution, and scientific medicine. Thus, the work of localizationists was closely followed by academic audiences in many disciplines. Scientists and nonscientists alike expected a definitive resolution to problems that had been debated for centuries by philosophers and theologians.

Yet in the face of this optimism, localizationist physicians and physiologists mapping the brain faced constant, severe uncertainties, most of which were never resolved. How did the different kinds of daily uncertainty in the laboratory, at the bedside, or in the surgical theater become transformed into the unquestioned premises of the map of localized functions?

Scientists and Uncertainty

Adherents to a scientific theory or perspective continually reconcile or absorb anomalous material into its basic tenets. This has been called "unfalsifiability" or "disconfirmation bias" by some, and this absorption defines, in many ways, a Kuhnian paradigm (Lakatos and Musgrave 1970; Polanyi 1964; Holton 1973). The persistence of belief, in the face of anomalies or contradictions, is one dependent variable of a sociological process that transforms local work uncertainties into more widely held theoretical certainties.

In his analysis of scientific change, Kuhn (1970) posited that a "critical mass" of anomalies eventually forces paradigmatic change. Scientists proceed with business as usual, despite anomalous events that are potentially threatening to that routine. As a paradigm shift occurs and science moves from "normal" to "revolutionary," anomalies come to have a different meaning.

By contrast with Kuhn, my analysis here shows that the practical negotiations with and about anomalous events are constitutive of science at every level of organization. There is a complex interplay between long- and short-term scientific goals, proximate and distant audiences, and specific historical circumstances in producing major conceptual shifts. And this occurs continually and routinely in science, not under special conditions of change. Perhaps by understanding the ways in which localizationist researchers managed these many contingencies, we can begin to better understand how and why "unfalsifiable" commitments are made and how the exigencies of daily scientific work become transformed or absorbed into widely accepted truths.

Scientists constantly face uncertainty. Their experimental materials are recalcitrant; their organizational politics are precarious; they may not know whether a given technique was correctly applied or interpreted; and they must often rely on observations made in haste or by unskilled assistants. As many observers of science have noted, these contingencies rarely appear in published descriptions of scientific work (Dewey et al. 1917). Recent studies of the path from laboratory to published work have shown that the transmogrification and deletion of uncertainties trace the birth of a "fact" (Latour 1980; Knorr-Cetina 1981; Zenzen and Restivo 1982; Law 1985; Latour and Bastide 1986). Bruno Latour and Steve Woolgar's *Laboratory Life* (1979) documents in some detail how scientists transform everyday uncertainties into facts via "deletion of modalities" and progressive reification. That is, statements that were once modified or qualified ("it appears that," or "our tentative conclusion is that") become unqualified truth ("it is the case that," or simply "it is"). Michael Lynch's study of art and artifact in the laboratory in the administration of neurobehavioral tests demonstrates a similar progression; his focus is on the negotiation and channeling between scientists in developing classes of truth (1982, 1985; see also Garfinkel, Lynch, and Livingston 1981).

One major thrust of this research thus far has been to document the presentation of data, from observation to publication, as increasingly certain. The published data reveal, rather than hint at; articles state, rather than guess at; and subjects line up docilely to be counted. Their attempts to run away, their individual differences, and their resistance to the experiments are erased from the public record. These observations about the deletion of uncertainty have added valuable insight about the process of conducting science (Collins 1975, Williams and Law 1980, Woolgar 1980, Pinch 1981, and Callon, Law, and Rip 1986 document a similar process in a variety of scientific settings.) However, the deletions have rarely been described with reference to the details of *both* large-scale organizational/political factors and hands-on laboratory or clinical practice; descriptions have also tended to focus on single cases or lines of work.

Studies such as *Laboratory Life* richly document the reduction of complex laboratory results into the vastly more simplified formats of formal scientific publications. Several aspects of this transformation might be further explored to understand multiple-site, long-term changes. These unexplored contingencies are central to understanding the transformation of uncertainty from the laboratory to larger-scale and longer-term enterprises, be they "paradigms," schools of thought, or laws of nature. Among these contingencies are the long-term effects of *combining* multiple sorts of evidence (for example, of clinical evidence with basic research) and the cumulative creation of certainty from multiple lines of evidence.

The *varieties* of uncertainty faced by scientists have received little attention: for example, the differences between the uncertainty introduced by a new and unfamiliar piece of technology and that introduced by lack of clarity about the meaning of a basic term. It is in understanding the practices by which uncertainties are resolved that the sociology of science can make a real contribution to the old philosophical discussions of generalizability and falsifiability. Scientists are intelligent problem-solvers, and their methods are sensible in the context of their constraints and resources. Scientists manage uncertainty by the successful negotiation of myriad obstacles and the articulation of difficulties present in any work site. These can include moral, political, and managerial pressures, design complexities, access to research materials, information, and skill, all of which may be recalcitrant or scarce. Scientists develop certainty with reference to larger spheres of work and longer time frames: multiple sites and audiences, perhaps other disciplines and institutions, and debates with opposing schools of thought.

I have interviewed many scientists who characterize the management of uncertainty as "not really science" (and with pejoratives including "mere administrative work," "dirty politics," "bean-counting," "mere logistics," and even "sociology"). *Real* science, on the other hand, means contributing to Truth *despite* these local "glitches" or "kludges." But certainty develops as local contingencies are jettisoned, minimized, distributed, or otherwise resolved. Taking care of local uncertainty, including its transformation to certainty, is not incidental; it is central to research organization, despite its deprecation by scientists.

We cannot assume that strategies for uncertainty management are universal or that uncertainty itself is monolithic. The conditions and responses to those strategies presented here are not historically or situationally invariant, nor do the types represent an exhaustive list. I hope this model for the complex transformation of daily uncertainty into larger historical contexts of action will be modified and extended.[1] At times, political uncertainty will drive a problem-solving enterprise; at other times, diagnostic uncertainty prevents work from proceeding until it has been resolved.

This analysis falls between several disciplinary divides. Medical sociologists have written about the uncertainties of diagnosis or medical training, but they have scarcely dealt with those of basic medical research (but see Clarke 1985).[2] Sociologists of science, as noted above, have elaborated individual-site or line-of-work uncertainties and their resolution, but rarely have they studied multiple-site, multiple-line transformations. And, in medical history, transformation of uncertainty has often been simply analyzed as "progress"—uncertainties dealt with purely as technical discoveries or difficulties to be overcome.

Although nineteenth-century localizationist medical research may appear to be remote from modern investigation, in fact the diagnostic, taxonomic, organizational, and technical uncertainties it faced are in no way analytically distinct from those faced by other scientists. A taxonomist facing a fuzzy species identification question (Hull 1976, 1982; Volberg 1983b), a paleontologist with a sparse fossil record, an astronomer with a foggy lens, or a maverick physiologist unable to obtain funding will be familiar with the types of uncertainties described herein and perhaps also with their transformations.

Types of Uncertainty

Localizationist workers in the several lines of work I examined all experienced great uncertainty. *Taxonomic* uncertainty arose as they tried to develop classification systems (for example, what kind of thing was epilepsy?). *Diagnostic* uncertainty appeared as they attempted to apply classifications (did this patient *have* epilepsy?). *Organizational* uncertainty arose in the course of creating or maintaining divisions of labor, collaborations, and alliances. *Technical* uncertainty was created by the vicissitudes of instruments and experimental materials.

In the face of the neat, familiar maps of the brain that have become standard since the days of Ferrier and Jackson, it is perhaps hard to imagine the initial uncertainty they faced. Nature is recalcitrant and elusive. Many of the physiological events the localizationists investigated were rare, unstable, episodic, or self-reversing; many of them seemed to begin in one place and spread to another. Materials, including cadavers, animals, and brains, were difficult to obtain or preserve and were often expensive. In addition, the topography of individual brains and nervous systems varies enormously from subject to subject; researchers were establishing anatomical baselines for measurement at the same time as they were trying to localize phenomena. For a fascinating discussion of the history of uncertainty and disagreement about the location of Wernicke's Region, see the discussion in Bogen and Bogen 1976. They note that many researchers over the years represented the region in vastly different ways. I sometimes think of them as explorers in a shifting, ill-marked terrain, inventing compasses as they traveled.

Organizational conditions added to the uncertainties of physio-

logical investigation. Financial insecurity, poor communication between investigators, and poor management-staff relations were some
of the contributing factors at the organizational level. Specialists and
nonspecialists handled many of the same cases from which data were
drawn; however, this meant that standards of data collection and
treatment varied even within the same case. And, always in the background, antivivisectionists threatened to bring *all* physiological research to a halt.

Despite these conditions, localizationist researchers persisted in
transforming uncertainty into fact. Confusion about categories gave
way to smoothly formed atlases of function, ideal types that could explain much in a general way. Diagnostic uncertainty gave way to elaborated taxonomies and a repertoire of more or less definitive symptoms. Organizational uncertainties formed the basis for development
of specific markets, specializations, and alliances. Technical uncertainty was handled by cutting problems into small pieces, standardizing techniques, and jettisoning intractable anomalies. I examine
each of these transformations in detail below.

Taxonomic Uncertainty

Classification was a difficult problem with nervous diseases—
symptom configurations both overlapped and were highly variable
within groups. In addition, brain tumors and some nervous diseases
were quite rare. Arriving at a "typical picture" of a given neurological
disease was particularly complicated for these reasons.

From the early part of the period under study (roughly 1860–1870),
Queen Square admitted patients by symptom: seizures, paralysis, and
the inability to speak were the most common. Physicians there were
faced with the problem of constructing disease categories from a heterogeneous patient group, such as those with tuberculosis, neurasthenia, syphilis, stroke, tumors, lesions, deficiency diseases, and lead
poisoning. Symptoms could also be transient within groups: patients
would sometimes relearn or reproduce lost functions after damage or
with slow tumor growth. The episodic nature of symptoms, their
transience, and the overlaps between disease categories made finding
a typical picture extremely difficult.

Stephen Paget, discussing a speech by the Queen Square surgeon

Horsley, said: "He spoke of the confusion of theories of epilepsy, and of the vague phrases in which the disease was described" (1919: 122–23). From ancient times, epilepsy had been a medical and social mystery; it had many forms, perhaps constituted many different diseases, and certainly had many different catalysts (Waller 1882; Temkin 1945; Rosen 1968). Brain tumors were equally vague and multiform. Symptoms included those common to many diseases: nausea, headache, dizziness, vision difficulties. Furthermore, because brain tumors were rare, each case's individual quirks loomed large in constructing taxonomies. Comparative samples were impossible.

Taxonomic uncertainty in the physiological work of the 1870's and 1880's arose from similar conditions. The physiologist's mandate was to discover the bases of nervous function, primarily by reproducing human disease conditions in healthy animals. Taxonomic uncertainty arose in part from uncertainty about whether and to what extent experimental ablations or lesions could be compared with human diseases. Could using animals of a different species be used to construct the same categories? Were areas impaired by tumor comparable to those eroded by tubercular lesions? The attempt to construct clear categories was clouded by these problems of comparability. The clinical neurologist Gowers, for example, noted in an exasperated tone that: "No symptoms have been observed in man corresponding to the functional centres that you often see marked on these convolutions in diagrams of the human brain, to which they have been transferred from the brains of monkeys" (1885: 170).

A clean link between cortical areas and the resulting movements or dysfunctions in experimental animals was requisite for an unambiguous taxonomy. Uncertainty arose, however, as scientists applied techniques designed to elicit these responses. For example, Ferrier's early research attempted to map the movements of muscles following extremely precise application of electrical current to parts of the cerebral cortex in monkeys. Yet electrical current spreads; it cannot be contained in one area. Critics attributed many of the muscle movements he found in his early (1870's) research to diffusion of current over the surface of the brain or into deeper structures. They claimed that his results did not indicate localized areas, but rather reflected a procedural artifact (Burdon-Sanderson 1873–74; Dodds 1877–78; Rabagliati 1879). A similar spreading effect was observed in surgical procedures where infection or hemorrhage distorted the boundaries of the areas under investigation. Diffusionists made similar criticisms of these findings.

A lack of information or scarcity of experimental material also contributed to taxonomic uncertainty. Neurosurgery was a new specialty, actually a new possibility, in the 1880's. There were few practicing neurosurgeons during the entire last quarter of the nineteenth century. Neurosurgeons working on research problems or on improvements in clinical treatments had few colleagues with whom they could compare cases. From 1886 to 1891, for example, Horsley remained the only neurosurgeon at Queen Square (Jefferson 1960). Physicians there saw patients only one or two times per week, and patients could have many seizures per day. This division of labor was therefore significant in augmenting uncertainty.

Because of the antivivisection restrictions (strictly enforced after the 1876 Cruelty to Animals Act), surgeons also had difficulty obtaining animals for experiments, which had to be performed on licensed animals during restricted hours. Similarly, pathologists had difficulty obtaining materials. Relatives were reluctant to give permission to do postmortems—the concept of autopsy was not widely honored outside the medical community. And if permission were given, work had to proceed quickly and discreetly.

Horsley, for example, in order to obtain bodies for postmortems, made an alliance with the porter at the mortuary of the hospital where he had his first job in the early 1880's. He removed—in essence, stole—organs from dead bodies, with the compliance of this porter (Lyons 1966). There was no other way for him to obtain a steady supply of cadavers for research. Yeo, a physician at Queen Square, remarked that the postmortem examination of the brain of a tumor patient "had to be performed hastily, and under difficulties which precluded the possibility of a detailed examination of that organ being made" (1878: 275). In that same case report, he complained of his difficulty in convincing the family to give permission for the patient to have a brain operation. The patient kept going into remission, apparently obviating the need for such high-risk surgery.

Clinical and basic uncertainties overlapped here. If a patient died from an operation for which the family finally gave its reluctant permission, the family was then naturally reluctant to allow a postmortem. Even where the family did give permission for an autopsy, there were difficulties. Ringrose Atkins noted the following:

The spinal cord presented nothing abnormal to the naked eye. Portions of the brain and spinal cord were placed aside for future microscopical examination, but unfortunately got spoiled in preparing, during my absence from home, therefore I regret that, so far as the microscopical examination could have thrown further light on the case, the report is imperfect. (1878: 413–14)

Bennett, in the same year, noted great difficulty in retrieving the brain of a dead patient who had had a cerebral tumor, since it had been accidentally thrown away. Ferrier (1879) described similar difficulties.

Because of a lack of comparative data, it was impossible for these researchers clearly to characterize the components of a "typical" disease. The autopsy report on the brain of a dog observed by Ferrier's partner, Yeo, discussed this as a major problem:

A great deal remains to be done before the brains of different dogs can be at all accurately divided into corresponding areas; for it is clear that some variation in the real position of the fissures might still take place. . . . In any case the division of the cortex into areas is only approximate, for it is impossible to say [to] which of the boundary convolutions the cortex at the bottom of the fissure belongs, if indeed it does belong to one more than to the other; this can only be done when we find a difference in histological structure. But what I wish to point out is that if the apparently corresponding fissures do not run along corresponding lines of the cortex, experiments made on the functions of the parts of the cortex in one dog afford very inadequate data for mapping out the cortex of the brains of other dogs, and *a fortiori* of mapping out the cortex of the brains of other animals. (Langley 1883–84: 250; see also Klein, Langley, and Schafer 1883–84)

The principal responses to taxonomic uncertainty were to standardize the formats in which data were recorded or to find exemplary cases that would typify categories. Taxonomies could then be refined by comparing data against ideal types, discarding "accidents" or anomalous findings.

One type of clinical information that lent itself easily to the development of comparative categories was the temporal progression of symptoms through the body. For example, epileptic seizures could start in a fingertip and move up an arm, gradually involving a whole side of the body. Or, as a tumor grew, symptoms could be observed spreading from one region to another. Beginning in the 1860's, doctors, patients, kin, and attendants tracked this "march" of symptoms and collected data that would transform them into taxonomies.

As localization theory gained prominence, Jackson (and, later, Ferrier) linked these symptoms with specific areas of the brain, sorting seizures by *region* of origin, sometimes linked with brain tumors. After about 1875, and with increasing refinement, physicians used this method to classify epilepsy and the location of tumors causing epileptic seizures.

To facilitate the recording of clinical data, these early neurologists created preprinted forms they called "fits sheets" for recording epileptic seizures. These sheets allowed patients, families, or medical attendants to check off information on the forms about the location of a spasm and the temporal particulars. The forms helped sift through the various aspects of taxonomic uncertainty in several ways: they provided a checklist so that categories did not have to be regenerated in order to obtain a natural history of each seizure, and record-making was sped up so that more information within a narrow range could be gathered.

The forms were also a source of an important transformation of uncertainty. Fuzzy intercategory data were ruled out by the checklist nature of the sheet, forcing observations into a clear taxonomy. Horsley's casebook (1904) contains the following directions to patients: "State very clearly on which side the movement commences, and whether it is confined to that side or spreads to the opposite side." (Although forms were an important tool in standardizing taxonomies, they did not ensure certainty at the level of data collection. I saw many forms that had been partially or vaguely filled out. Patients often left blanks and used phrases such as: "Yes, no, ? . . . "; "Feels lethargic"; "Twitches all over"; "I don't know"; or "Felt poorly" [National Hospital Records 1870–1901].)[3]

Physiologists, too, attempted to standardize their procedures, materials, and protocols in order to obtain unambiguous data for establishing taxonomies. After Ferrier's early experiments, for example, he began using preprinted outline sketches of brains to label functional areas according to muscle reactions (Ferrier 1873–1883).

Another response to taxonomic uncertainty was to find exemplary, unambiguous cases of particular diseases. Such cases were often written up in the medical journals or presented in medical classrooms: the "perfect" tumor demonstrated a localized function, or a "classic" case of epilepsy. In filtering for textbook cases, clinicians were able to establish taxonomies without the uncertainty created by overlapping symptom boundaries or individual differences (Jones 1899, 1959). Although the uncertainties would reappear at the diagnostic stage, the fundamental structure of medical work depended on clear taxonomies, not clear diagnosis (see, for example, Lester King's discussion [1982] of the differences between nosology [taxonomy] and diagnosis).

Diagnostic Uncertainty

Diagnostic uncertainty arose when investigators attempted to fit a particular case into their taxonomies. It is fascinating to observe here how taxonomic and diagnostic uncertainty interact: if we are not sure what a given disease should typically look like, how do we tell if someone has it? If symptoms are highly variable or hard to identify, how do we create a typical picture?

Diseases of the nervous system are very labile and are rarely limited either in their location or in their effects on the organism (Gowers 1885; Bramwell 1888; Paget 1919:180–81). The tumors found by investigators did not grow in neat patterns or conform to topographical diagrams of the brain. Instead, they expanded across the analytic boundaries created by researchers. They not only spread to different areas of the cortex but also descended (or originated) in the lower parts of the brain, thus violating the often fragile boundaries of functional neurological theories. Tumors and other nervous system disorders also had multifarious side effects. These included increases in intracranial pressure, scar tissue, and changes in vein growth and other circulatory patterns. Infections, as a result of surgery or of necrotic abscesses, were common, uncontrollable, and occult in their effects. Infections that resulted from brain operations (such as brain fungus and meningitis) were common.

Individuals also produced widely varying "pictures" of different nervous system diseases, adding another potent source of uncertainty.

Thomas Buzzard, for example, described one patient with a huge tumor who appeared entirely unaffected by it. Upon the patient's death, Buzzard noted in a puzzled tone: "It is *remarkable* that a person suffering from so extensive and grave an intracranial lesion should have been able to enjoy a long day's hunting within a week of his death" (1881: 132).

Both surgeons and neurologists also faced uncertainty because many diseases shared symptoms with brain tumors: lead poisoning, thyroid diseases, muscular dystrophy, and so on. Among these diseases was advanced syphilis. As with brain tumors, tertiary syphilis could cause paralysis, epileptic-like seizures, and blindness. Conservative physicians wanted *all* patients with these symptoms to undergo a prophylactic course of treatment for syphilis before even considering a diagnosis of brain tumor. This meant a wait of at least six weeks, a period that was often decisive in the clinical trajectory of a tumor patient.

Surgeons and neurologists bitterly fought this conservatism, but it continued to interfere with swift diagnosis and treatment until the Wasserman test (a swift, simple test) was developed in 1908 (de-Watteville 1881; Cushing 1905; Horsley 1906). This was long after the basic tenets of localizationism were established. A letter from Gowers (a neurologist) to Horsley (a surgeon) attests to some of the difficulties: "Possible syphilis and urgency to act as *soon* as ever the *absence* of result from treatment is *just* definite enough. I hear you think it is very likely a large tumour. I suppose you will do the second part, here, as soon as is proper. Can you tell me when?" (Lyons 1965: 263–64).

Surgery and autopsy provided confirmation of diagnostic puzzles and thus were important tools in the gradual reduction of diagnostic and taxonomic uncertainty. There were also many other responses to diagnostic uncertainty, several of which involved postponing diagnostic decisions or substituting unclear neurological information from more certain realms.

At admission, patients with seizures, aphasia, or paralysis were provisionally diagnosed by physicians and treated with a wide variety of remedies. The provisional categories were often refined according to surgical or pathological data obtained after the patient's death. Thus the immediate diagnostic uncertainty was often managed by simple postponement. Postmortem or physiological evidence became part of the body of taxonomic, not diagnostic, data. Curiously, therefore, diagnostic data were often not immediately helpful with daily clinical problems. The validation of many diagnostic classifications could only be proven after patients died, or by indirect inference. The diagnostic uncertainty, then, was temporally segmented within the workplace (for a general discussion of this, see Davis 1956; Hougland and Shepard 1980).

Diagnostic uncertainty in neurology was rarely addressed directly in terms of diagnostic validation of neurological exam techniques or of better testing equipment. Instead, neurologists focused on expanding and refining taxonomies. The elaboration of the familiar reflex-test battery of modern neurology, for example, was a major concern at Queen Square in the late nineteenth century. During the latter part of this period, neurologists relied heavily on a combination of general taxonomies and post hoc anatomical validation to resolve puzzles posed by diagnosis (Hunter and Hurwitz 1961).

Neurologists often hired diagnostic and taxonomic consultants. For instance, Felix Semon, an ear, nose, and throat doctor, was consulted on a regular basis to see if those patients unable to speak suffered organic disease of the larynx. His job was to rule out that form of disease before others hypothesized a brain tumor. Similarly, ophthalmologists were often consulted for patients with vision loss.

Treatment was also organizationally segmented. Lower-status physicians or attendants gave electrical treatment; nurses and attendants administered massages and bromides. Neurologists were thus free to concern themselves with refining research taxonomies and with public lecturing, teaching, and writing articles about diseases of the nervous system (Holmes 1954). This separation of care and diagnosis made both more certain in the short run. Attendants and consultants could screen out complications and side effects. They collected data that would fit within the categories represented on the forms. From this information base, neurologists were able to cull unambiguous cases for publication and demonstration.

Another response of neurologists to diagnostic uncertainty was to seek *pathognomonic signs*—that is, signs that uniquely indicate a certain disease. Many disease signs could provide ambiguous information. An impaired knee reflex, for example, could potentially indicate any of several different conditions. Neurologists initially thought they had discovered a pathognomonic sign for brain tumors: optic neuritis. This is an inflammation of the optic nerve that is directly visible to the doctor on physical examination. In 1871 Jackson said that optic neuritis was the most common ophthalmological condition in cerebral disease. By 1877 he was convinced that, without ophthalmology, methodical investigation of diseases of the nervous system was not merely difficult but impossible (Spillane 1981: 354–58). In the same vein, Gowers wrote to Horsley about 1894 that the absence of optic neuritis was sufficient to rule out a brain tumor: "No headache no optic neuritis. What more wd you want before operating? Of course op.n. would suffice but one can't propose it yet to friends though I have to a cousin doctor" (Lyons 1965: 263).

Yet even this seemingly clear purchase on diagnostic uncertainty was to prove tenuous. By 1906 Horsley was writing on the complexity of optic neuritis as a symptom. Optic disks swell and atrophy over the course of a disease and prove elusive indicators at different disease stages (Spillane 1981: 412). Spillane describes Gowers's reaction to the problem:

Optic neuritis was *the* ocular lesion in intracranial tumour; it was present in about four-fifths of cases. But it did not seem to be related to the site, size, or nature of the tumour, or even to its rate of growth. Optic neuritis was not a constantly associated condition in the history of a cerebral tumour; it was a transient event. A tumour might exist and cause symptoms for years before optic neuritis was produced. . . . The atrophy left by optic neuritis . . . could not always be diagnosed with certainty. (1981: 360)

Finally, clinicians responding to diagnostic uncertainty were forced to treat each patient with a wide variety of therapies. In the absence of simple testing procedures or pathognomonic signs, they had only the hope that by giving patients a number of different therapies, one would succeed. Patients at Queen Square were massaged, electrified, and given steam baths and mud plaster, potassium bromide, "metallotherapy" (an obscure treatment that involved placing metal disks over different parts of the body), and even leeches (Bennett 1878; Urquhart 1878; Buzzard casebook 1901, National Hospital Records; Rawlings 1913).

Organizational Uncertainty

Organizational uncertainty arose when information was lost or trapped owing to the local division of labor or the circumstances of alliances and collaborations. There were often gaps in communication between doctors and patients, between physicians and surgeons, or between care-taking staff and management. Political uncertainty also arose from the precarious nature of relationships with research and clinical sponsors, funding negotiations, conflict about professional status, and debates with scientists of opposing schools of thought.

Although the specialized nature of the hospital at Queen Square created research opportunities, it increased uncertainties in the relationships between specialists and general practitioners. Nonspecialists often did not know how to diagnose nervous diseases—even specialists had only just developed their tests in the 1870's and 1880's.

In part because of the lack of knowledge about nervous system diseases among the general medical community, patients frequently did not get referred to Queen Square until the advanced stages of their diseases. The referrals would thus come after more subtle symptoms had been missed, or after patients had undergone ineffective treatments elsewhere. For instance, one casebook of Ferrier's from 1894 records that a patient with a cerebral tumor had been discharged from the army several months before his admission to Queen Square with a diagnosis of "debility from climate and military service" (National Hospital Records). Here there was an interaction between lack of specialist knowledge, organizational uncertainty, and diagnostic uncertainty.

As I discussed in Chapter 2, British surgeons were fighting during this period for equal status with physicians. Although surgeons had achieved nominal equality with physicians in professional associations by the 1880's, there were still significant inequities. Physicians controlled most access to patients, and surgeons had to bargain with them to obtain cases. Thus relationships between physicians and surgeons were a continuing source of uncertainty and antagonism.

This rivalry framed some of the later developments in localization theory. Neurology came to be equated with research and management of the problems of the "mind," particularly with classifying its disturbances into a localized taxonomy. The mind could be reached, it was thought, by gentle means: reflex tests, psychological examination, observation. The mental taxonomies so developed were verified by other lines of work via more anatomical methods. Some of the subtle philosophical commitments to visions of mind/brain interaction came to be built into the very organization of clinical work practiced by localizationists. (This is discussed in some detail in Chapter 7.) The fashion in which uncertainties were managed in neurology and other lines of work solidified this organization of work. A division arose between lines of work that emphasized diagnosis and those that employed manual/anatomical skills, and as time went on this division was institutionalized in both organizational practice and philosophical commitment.

The record-keeping at Queen Square reflected the inequities between physicians and surgeons. I had some trouble locating Horsley's casebooks and was told that surgical cases were maintained separately from medical cases. After searching through the entire hospital, I finally found that Horsley's case notes (like the notes of nurses, attendants, and house physicians) had been appended to those of the physician in cases requiring brain, spinal cord, or nervous system operations. The physicians' names were stamped in gold on the leatherbound volumes, and Horsley's name was to be found only in his signature at the bottom of the surgical reports.

Letters between Gowers and Horsley also reflect a tense situation, in which communication and cooperation were often tenuous. In one case, a patient grew much worse because Gowers could not locate Horsley to consult him about operating. The letters, as well as medical articles from the time, also complain of the negative attitude of many patients toward brain surgery (Lyons 1965).

The fact that the need for brain surgery was not immediately apparent to the general medical profession contributed to the political uncertainty surrounding localizationism. Surgeons and localizationist neurologists had first to convince the medical community that brain surgery was *possible* and, once possible, prudent. It was perhaps helpful that there were no effective alternatives for tumor patients. Neurologists had not developed effective treatments for such diseases (Cushing 1913). As Horsley grimly stated:

As in all special branches of medicine and surgery which are in a process of evolution, it is not easy to assign credit or blame when the course of treatment pursued is respectively successful or unsuccessful; but so long as our powers of diagnosis remain as imperfect as they are so long will the vulgar error of regarding surgical treatment as a *dernier ressort* be committed. This question, namely, When should medicinal treatment be given up and operative treatment substituted? has been raised again and again and hotly discussed in connexion with many diseases. (1906: 411)

And Cushing asked rhetorically: "For what eager student of medicine can face without dismay the 'poverty of therapy' that characterizes the present day, and which is emphasized more especially in the neurological clinic, which stands largely on the therapeutic tripod of iodine, bromide, and electricity?" (1905: 78).

The formation of neurosurgery from neurology and surgery gave neurology claim to a unique treatment for hitherto-untreatable cases, and in turn it provided surgeons with a theoretical base for localizationist therapies (Cushing 1920, 1935; Spillane 1981: 398). This had the gradual effect of reducing organizational uncertainty, perhaps at the expense of taxonomic and diagnostic uncertainty, as the neurosurgeon Cushing lucidly described:

The neurologist spends days or weeks in working out the presumable location and nature of, let us say, a cerebral tumor. An operator is called in; he has little knowledge of maladies of this nature and less interest in them, but is willing to undertake the exploration. The supposed site of the growth is marked out for him on the scalp by the neurologist; and he proceeds to trephine. The dura is opened hesitatingly; the cortex is exposed, and too often no tumor is found. The operator's interest ceases with the exploration, and for the patient the common sequel is a hernia, a fungus cerebri, meningitis, and death. (1905: 78)

Other kinds of organizational uncertainty in clinical work arose from management/staff conflicts in the hospital. At Queen Square there was continual friction among the hospital administrator, the board of governors, and the doctors. One bone of contention was control of admissions. Physicians demanded exclusive jurisidiction in admitting patients, especially for acute, scientifically interesting cases. Hospital administrators and governors, on the other hand, wanted to control admissions themselves, for financial and political reasons. The tradeoffs here were fairly straightforward: when administrators controlled admissions, physicians never knew when there would be an empty bed, or with what illnesses they would be confronted. When physicians controlled them, income for the hospital was unpredictable (Rawlings 1913; Holmes 1954).

The major political uncertainty for physiology was a lack of independent funding or institutional security, which was in part because of opposition from antivivisectionists and in part because of the general lack of British resources available for basic physiological research (French 1975; Geison 1978). Foster described the antivivisection situation in his 1881 inaugural address to the Physiology Section of the International Medical Congress in London:

Our science has been made the subject of what the highest legal authority stated in the House of Lords to be a *penal act*. We are liable at any moment in our inquiries to be arrested by legal prohibitions, we are hampered by licenses and certificates. When we enter upon any research we do not know how far we may go before we have to crave permission to proceed, laying bare our immature ideas before those who are, in our humble opinion, unfit to judge them; and we often find our suit refused. (MacCormac 1881: 218)

The pressure for localizationist researchers to resolve all sorts of uncertainties and to present clinically useful results is palpable in this address. Some of the organizational strategies used to reduce uncertainty are described below.

Dividing groups and treatment responsibilities. Organizational uncertainty between physicians and surgeons was handled in part by segregating patients with operable tumors from those with less obvious problems. Physicians submitted their diagnoses to surgeons for review for possible brain surgery; they then provided neurological information that might help surgeons locate tumors. Other patients were cared for exclusively by physicians and support staff (Lyons 1965).

Focus on clinical impact. Localizations met institutional precariousness with a conservative, anatomically oriented approach that was geared toward clinical validation. Physiologists did struggle to gain a separate institutional base from medicine, but in England this was successful only much later. Experimenters used clinical successes to validate localization theory and then used the theory to legitimate vivisection, as discussed in the following chapter (Geison 1978: 27–28).

Crichton-Browne, a founding editor of the localizationist journal *Brain*, wrote this letter to the London *Times* in 1884:

Sire, – While the Bishop of Oxford and Professor Ruskin were, on somewhat intangible grounds, denouncing vivisection at Oxford last Tuesday afternoon, there sat at one of the windows of the Hospital for Epilepsy and Paralysis, in Regent's Park, in an invalid chair, propped up with pillows, pale and care-worn, but with a hopeful smile on his face, a man who could have spoken a really pertinent word upon the subject, and told the right rev. prelate and great art critic that he owed his life, and his wife and children their rescue from bereavement and penury, to some of these experiments on living animals which they so roundly condemned. The case of this man has been watched with intense interest by the medical profession, for it is of a unique description, and inaugurated a new era in cerebral surgery. (Spillane 1981: 398)

In banding together to form the Physiological Society for the purposes of combating antivivisection, physiologists (who were often physicians) formed powerful cross-disciplinary alliances. This had the effect of linking provivisection advocates with physiology in a very general fashion (Sharpey-Schafer 1927).

Focus on details of individual cases. The organizational uncertainties presented by pathological work required coping with research situations in which materials were scarce—and in which obtaining any materials could be a source of considerable stigma (if not actually criminal). Although postmortem work came to be routine after the turn of the century, it was still often difficult, for organizational reasons, to obtain good comparative data. Pathologists were forced to take samples when and where they could and to preserve them as well as they could. This had the direct effect of reinforcing a focus on the minutiae of individual cases, especially of brain tumors, rather than on the issues arising from comparative work. Pathologists relied on the case-by-case microscopic examination of brains and nervous tissue. This organization of work was important, because uncertainties were resolved using a combination of clinical, physiological, and pathological data. Potentially contradictory evidence from broad ranges of pathological data did not appear until much later in the course of localization theory. By the time it did, the adherents of the theory were firmly ensconced in their scientific places.

Technical Uncertainty

Technical uncertainty developed as a result of inadequate tools or ambiguous information about techniques. The experimental subjects used by Ferrier and others included dogs, rabbits, monkeys, birds, and even jackals. Technical uncertainty arose from difficulties with subjects, equipment, and procedures, including the lack of standard measurement techniques.

Many of Ferrier's exemplary experiments consisted of opening the skull of an animal and systematically applying electrical current to a sequence of minute cortical regions. He then recorded subsequent muscle movements. The points of application were carefully numbered. If the animal survived surgery, the next step was to attempt to identify accurately the various brain centers. Uncertainty arose in attempting to account for individual animal anatomical variations and to control the amount and kind of electrical current. These became major sources of artifact and potential error (Burdon-Sanderson 1873–74; Dodds 1877–78; Duret 1878).

The difficulty of working with reacting subjects, particularly monkeys, is vividly conveyed by Ferrier's laboratory notebooks. His notes were often written in an obviously hasty, shaky hand as he tried to record minute-by-minute events in the laboratory. The pages of several notebooks are spattered with blood stains. Ferrier noted that the monkeys were often "mischievous," hostile, or affectionate and that they were constantly trying to run away from him, climb up his pant legs, bite, or scratch. In Ferrier's words:

Apparently monkey disinclined to move. Could see somewhat as he when making a push away from being pursued did not knock except occasionally. . . . Difficult to say whether right extended or not as being disinclined to move it—at any rate we had few methods of testing. . . . After this we tried hard to get the bandage off the left eye. Was very unwilling to move at all. When kicked would run against anything. Taken into the other room. Sat still with head down. Would not respond to when called. Gave him a piece of cracker and he put it in his mouth. Took him back into laboratory. Got quite still and grunted or made a rush anywhere when distracted. (Ferrier 1873–1883: January 5, 1875, MS246/5)

In addition to being reactive in a behavioral sense, the animals were physiologically fragile. Damage to animal subjects, including operative complications, was common. The notebooks record frequent accidental deaths in the laboratory from hemorrhage or chloroform overdose.

In 1873, at the time of Ferrier's initial experiments, antisepsis had not been accepted as standard even for human surgery, and many experimenters furthermore believed that animals were resistant to infection. They did not think it necessary to take precautions for animal operations (French 1975). A. Rabagliati, in describing the work of Hermann Munk, said that Munk "has not been able definitely to localize the representations, however, because all his animals died of most acute meningitis in his efforts to remove the surrounding centres" (1879: 537–38).

Two Italian localizationists, Luigi Luciani and Augusto Tamburini, criticized Ferrier for not accounting for the artifacts introduced by injury to experimental animals. They said, "It is impossible to have exactly similar conditions present, no account being taken of the amount of the haemorrhage, of the amount of injury suffered, of the exhaustion of the two animals compared, of the narcosis, and of the precise amount of the electrisation" (Rabagliati 1879: 532).

Where to place electrodes, how to make incisions, and how to create lesions and then control them were all problematic. Although many of these technical problems were either resolved or standardized by the turn of the century, others, such as control and specificity, remain important even today. Ferrier's notes (1873–1883) depict these difficulties:

No application could be made nor could the electrolisation be made to be localised.

This movement was very difficult to analyse as the brain very speedily lost its excitability.

Hard to distinguish where the electrodes were due to the bleeding. (August 8, 1874, MS246/2)

He spoke of animals exhausted, in states of stupor (December 1874, MS246/4). He poked and prodded the animals, gave them smelling salts and electrical shocks, and banged on the water pipes to see if they would react. An experiment in 1879 recorded an operation whose sequelae Ferrier was "not sure if existed before" (October 1879, MS246/7).

Investigators had several responses to these conditions, including attempts to standardize techniques, reduce problem scope, and point away from work uncertainties and toward theoretical validity. In response to technical uncertainties such as the diffusion of electrical current, or questions about the comparability of types of current, investigators eventually settled on one standard technique. Similarly, the notational conventions discussed above were in part an attempt to correct for technical variation in data recording. Arguments about ambiguities in technique resulted in the adoption of standard incisions and promoted the standard use of antiseptic procedures. Conventions for notating brain areas and current were adopted, and the types of animals used for experimentation became increasingly uniform.

The immediate scope of the problems addressed by localizationists tended to narrow, partially in response to technical uncertainties. Famous experiments by Charles Edward Beevor and Victor Horsley in the 1890's attempted precisely to chart minute regions of the cerebral cortex. The uncertainty created in trying to analyze larger areas was thus circumvented (Beevor and Horsley 1890, 1894).

But many of the technical uncertainties faced by localizationists were—and continued to be—uncontrollable. One response to this was to substitute theoretical validity for technical consistency, and in the process to jettison those anomalies that remained intractable. For example, localizationists commonly encountered the following anomaly: a lesion occurred in an area of the brain thought to be responsible for a function, but the function remained intact. Instead of abandoning either their techniques or their theories, they categorized these (frequent) incidents as exceptions. Discussions of the logical tenets of localization replaced discussions of technical insufficiency.

Compare, for example, two statements made by Ferrier in *The Functions of the Brain* (1876). On page 38 he noted the inseparability of parts of the brain and thus the insignificance of the anomaly; on page 148, however, he called into question the significance of his findings should this be the case. Yet the whole book is an unqualified argument for localizationism.

In reading through the notebooks and articles of the period, I repeatedly came upon the phrase "failure to localise" or qualifications such as the following: "Had a different system of partitioning the brain to that which I adopted been pursued, perhaps even more striking results would have been obtained, and certainly more trustworthy data would have been collected bearing upon the researches of Hitzig and Ferrier" (Crichton-Browne 1879: 65).

Summary of Uncertainties: Conditions and Responses

The local uncertainties faced by researchers included the conditions and responses summarized in Table 1. Despite the many local uncertainties they experienced, researchers were confident about the long-range global validity and reliability of their results. As Henry Head, a neurophysiologist from the generation following Ferrier's, described their outlook:

> All this school of observers believed that they could interpret the clinical manifestations directly in terms of anatomical paths and centres; each one added one or more cases to those that had already become classical. . . . It was an era of robust faith and nobody suggested that the clinical data might be insufficient for each precise localisation; still less could they believe that the conclusions reported by men of eminent good faith might be grossly inaccurate. (Head 1926: vol. 1, p. 57)

And Ferrier said, "In spite of innumerable attempts to degrade the grey matter of the brain and to exclude it from all share in the results, it may be regarded as established that its definite groups of cells yield definite effects always constant under a definite stimulation of whatever nature" (1878b: 131). Even Rawlings, the hospital administrator, seemed convinced of the certainty of localization of function:

> The structure and working of the brain had been laid bare, and the stupendous fact had been established that to each of the cerebral hemispheres were allotted functions distinct and separate. These enthusiasts, pursuing their investigations under discouraging conditions with an untiring patience which

TABLE I
Summary of Local Uncertainties

	Conditions	Responses
Taxonomy	Rarity of events Multiple effects from single causes Individual differences Materials difficult to obtain Instability of events (episodic, self-reversing, spreading) Partially available data Diverse populations for study Unclear boundaries of causal phenomena; lack of causal models Uncontrollable experimental conditions Lack of information for comparison	Order data sequentially or by spatial location Standardize Find exemplars—filter for clear-cut cases
Diagnosis	Labile and spreading symptoms and side effects Delayed information Individual differences	Segmentation of uncertainty Substitution of taxonomy for diagnosis Division of labor Search for pathognomonic signs Shotgun treatments
Organizational	Specialist/nonspecialist handling of the same cases Unequal status between investigators Poor management-staff relations Lack of funding, sporadic funding; lack of institutional security Delays and lack of communication between investigators	Division of data along political lines for clarity Division of labor along technical/substantive lines Observations limited to available materials Utilitarian emphasis on practical results
Technical	Reacting subjects Operative complications (experimental) Uncontrollable procedures Observational difficulties	Standardization of techniques and materials Standardization of observational techniques (forms) and protocols Observations down-focused to smaller areas Substitution of theoretical validity for technical consistency

SOURCE: Star 1985a: 406.

invested their intelligence with genius, demonstrated that every individual portion of the seemingly homogeneous organ was allotted its own particular task, and in response to the probing interrogation of science every fibre and filament of the complex structure yielded up the secret of its being. (1913: 121)

It would be simple to dismiss such claims as mere braggadocio or exaggeration without adequate substantive bases. But such an analysis is too simple as well as *ad hominem*. The general public and the medical and scientific worlds, not just the researchers involved (influenced by their intitial investments), claimed certainty for localizationist findings. The laboratories and procedures were under close public scrutiny. In no way did they employ procedures significantly different from those common in science then or now (Star 1983). The question, from a sociological and historical point of view, is then: How did the myriad workplace uncertainties become transformed into disciplinary certainty?

Creating and Maintaining Certainty

Several mechanisms were involved in the transformation of local uncertainty into global certainty at the institutional level. Several of these involved substitutions of various types; all were rooted in work organization and political contexts. The mechanisms of transformation included attributing certainty across disciplinary boundaries— that is, transferring uncertainties from one realm to another. Researchers also substituted types of evaluation of results in creating global certainty: they used operational, not technical or product-oriented, evaluations for technical failures.

In addition, the ideal types generated by the intersection of taxonomic and diagnostic uncertainties became transformed into theoretical goals. With the backing of research and institutional sponsors for those goals, researchers were able to jettison potentially crippling anomalies and minimize the significance of individual differences. Case results were generalized on an ad hoc basis, minimizing some of the effects of a lack of comparative data as well as the effects of anomalies in physiological research arising from experimental failures. In this mode, localizationists oscillated between clinical and basic concerns in applying evaluation criteria.

Finally, the bitter debate with diffusionists had the effect of polarizing the scientists involved and subsuming epistemological questions in favor of the immediacy of the debate. I discuss each of these transformations in turn below.

Attributing Certainty to Other Fields

Evidence for localization was collected from several areas. As these were joined to describe the same phenomenon in a general argument, local contingencies from one field became invisible. Researchers tended to attribute certainty to other fields: physiologists relied on clinical evidence to supplement their anomalous or uncertain results; pathologists turned to physiological evidence when they could not find clear postmortem evidence for discrete functional regions.

Because of the attribution of certainty across disciplinary lines, it was impossible for researchers to trace a simple *path* of uncertainty, response, or negotiation of anomalous results. Lines of evidence became tangled, both in publication and in demonstration, but there was no public way of verifying this or of realizing that it was happening, since the details of work were embedded in the local contexts. Several aspects of this are discussed in more detail in the following chapter.

Substituting Operational Evaluations for Technical Failures

Members of a profession often account for failures not as mistakes or threats to validity, but as processes that can only be understood by insiders. Rue Bucher and Joan Stelling call this the development of "vocabularies of realism" and note that it is an important aspect of professional socialization. Such substitutions appear as expressions, such as "the patient died but the operation was a success." Professionals focus on "doing one's best" and "recognition of limitation," sometimes by ignoring the actual outcome of a given procedure (Freidson 1970a; Bucher and Stelling 1973; Bosk 1979).

An example of the use of vocabularies of realism in place of technical failures is found in this report from a contemporary of Horsley's, who considered the fact that many of Horsley's operations were only partially successful and many were technically complete failures. This was a stage for surgery of the nervous system, he opined, and in his words we can see the amalgam of clinical and technical evaluation criteria:

> The problems were to localise a tumour accurately by clinical means, to verify that diagnosis by operation, remove the tumour if possible. Nobody else could have done any better than Horsley . . . and when one had seen a man carried into Queen Square comatose, had seen Horsley remove a tumour, and one had afterwards met the man travelling on the underground railway in perfectly good health, in spite of a large lacuna in the vault of his skull, one had to admit that a very remarkable thing had been done. (Jones 1946: 153)

The substitution of operational evaluations for strictly technical evaluations of outcomes helped to transform local clinical uncertainty to global certainty by focusing on the more certain aspects of localization theory and ignoring partial successes or gray areas.

Ideal-Type Substitution

There was a steady and urgent demand from medical researchers and clinicians for textbooks, atlases, and other representations with accurate, useable depictions of typical diseases of the nervous system. John D. Spillane (1981: 403) discusses the widespread adoption of Gowers's textbook of neurology ("the bible of neurology") as a turning point in the field. The textbook contained many such functional atlases. Ernest Jones's notes (1899) from his medical training at University College Hospital also indicated the desire for and dissemination of such information by Queen Square staff.

In the process of resolving taxonomic uncertainty, researchers thus created *typical* pictures of diseases that were eagerly adopted by the medical community. These representations included functional anatomical maps—such as maps that could indicate the anatomical point in the brain that was the source of loss of speech. These maps became substitutes, in the building of localization theory, for case data that contained irregular or anomalous findings. The demand for functional anatomical representations in medical education, diagnosis, and texts represented a market intolerant of ambiguity and of individual differences. The theory became unambiguously packaged into the atlas. The ideal types represented in such maps were presented as context-independent (that is, as *the* brain, not *a* brain).[4]

It was crucial that localizationists had the backing of sponsors who overlooked anomalies and even assisted in the process of deleting them. Ferrier, for example, was briefly sponsored by a small grant from the Royal Society to conduct his early experiments. When he submitted his original report in 1873–74 to the society, referees took care to check the numbered regions Ferrier claimed for given functions. They disagreed with his placement of some regions. Rolleston's referee report (1874) on the experiments contains the following passage:

I have however to say, with reference to certain statements made on pages 30– 32 of the paper, that I do not think Dr. Ferrier is quite right in saying that the parts of the brain indicated by him with the circles ⑨ and ⑩ as stated to have called forth movements of the tongue and mouth are really the homologues of this region in man which is the seat of lesion in the disease known as aphasia. The seat of this lesion I believe is seated some distance in front of this locality indicated in Dr. Ferrier's figure ii by the circles ⑨ and ⑩.

Rolleston went on to suggest that Ferrier change the location of the number in question on the diagram. He also noted that Ferrier's earlier paper reporting work done at West Riding had circles and numbers placed differently, and he suggested that Ferrier standardize the two sets of drawings. It is important to note here that the suggestion was to *standardize the diagrams*, not to redo the experiments in light of what might alternatively have been seen as inconsistent findings. Thus the substitution of a more general map for specific experimental findings helped to add a good deal of credibility to the localizationist enterprise; the report to the Royal Society was widely cited and held by many to be definitive evidence for localization of function.

Another example of this same process may be seen in the presentation of clinical results and the subsequent maps. Once a patient was diagnosed as having a brain tumor, neurologists tried to localize it. Localizations often failed. Ernst von Bergmann, in 1889, "was able to collect seven cases only in which a brain tumor had been diagnosed by neurological evidence, localized, and removed by operation" (Horrax 1952: 56).

In the casebooks at Queen Square, I discovered a tracing that Hor-

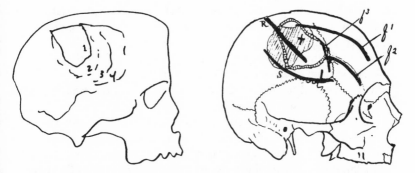

Fig. 1. On the left, a sketch made by surgeon Victor Horsley of progressive holes cut in a patient's skull while seeking to locate a tumor (Ferrier casebook 1886, National Hospital Records). Compare with sketch on the right showing similar holes (trephine openings) in the Knapp and Bradford operation discussed on p. 99 (1889: 328), for which successful localization was claimed. (The double line shows the trephine opening. The shaded portion shows the situation of the tumor. The cross shows the point marked before operating as the chief seat of the tumor. R = fissure of Rolando; S = fissure of Sylvius; f^1 and f^2 = first and second frontal sulci; f^3 = precentral sulcus.)

sley had made of his incision through the skull of a tumor patient. The drawing shows four separate openings, made successively in the operation as the tumor was repeatedly not found (see Figure 1). Ultimately, the hole encompassed nearly 25 percent of the entire skull area (Ferrier casebook, 1886, National Hospital Records; see also Beevor casebook, 1894, for a similar case in which no tumor was removed but a large amount of bone was removed in the search for it).

Yet these failures (anomalies and uncertainties) on the local level were not presented as invalidating evidence at a global level. Instead, clinical cures were used as evidence for the validity of localization theory, a process discussed in more detail in the following chapter.

Generalizing Case Results

The conventions for publishing medical research in the nineteenth century emphasized detailed case reports. Minute observations about patient progress, techniques, and medication were intermingled with basic research hypotheses in a fashion strange to modern eyes. Such reporting was an important contributor to the transformation of uncertainty from clinical sites. Localizationist researchers worked in several loosely coupled clinical and physiological research sites. Due to these reporting conventions, few controls (such as refereed papers or stringent methodological requirements) operated on the flow of information from research site to publication. Instead, information was added piecemeal to the corpus of medical research on localization, often in an inconsistent manner.

As a result, challenges to the validity of local findings tended to be distributed over the same scattered case results. Researchers assembled evidence from both clinical cases and physiological experiments in making their case for localization of function. In debates (both internal and external), evaluation would easily shift from clinical success to basic findings, in an unorganized fashion. The distributed nature of research organization, coupled with the conventions of medical writing, tended to deemphasize local uncertainties and failures. Thus two different pools of criteria for public success were available, whereas local failures went unreported.

Subsuming Epistemological Questions to Debates About Technique

Diffusionists denied that functions could be located in particular parts of the brain (see, for example, Brown-Séquard 1890b). Initially, localizationist writing was defensive in posture: much of the evidence collected to prove localization was directed toward making the negative case for diffusionism. This approach focused on arguments against the other position, not on establishing positive proof or elaborating positive arguments. Counterpoints to arguments raised from outside the localizationist research endeavor thus often served to bury local uncertainties.

Debates about technique and method did take place within the localizationist camp, however, and here it is important to understand that arguments within a position strengthen that position. For example, the more that localizationists argued with one another about *how* to do ablation experiments, the less salient the question of *whether* to do them became. Widespread or high-level uncertainties about the validity of localization itself became transformed into more manageable, lower-level concerns with technique. Debate, both within localizationist science and between camps, thus subsumed epistemological uncertainty.

Summary

Scientists work simultaneously in two incommensurable contexts: local organizational settings and national/international disciplines. In the local workplace, specific *actions* resolve uncertainty. These actions "satisfice," in Herbert Simon's terms—it is often too expensive, or simply impossible, to obtain all the information needed to act within the time during which the action is possible (Simon 1981).

Management of uncertainty in the local work setting is heuristic, often ad hoc, and tailored to cope with the material and political exigencies of the given context. Yet scientists also justify their actions to larger audiences as contributors to a discipline. The results that they publish in this context cannot, by convention, reflect much local contingency. One of the mandates of science is to create generalizable results, which are meant to be universal, and this mandate is often conflated with the deletion of local contingency. Balancing the two contexts results in a series of strategies through which scientists satisfy local constraints and create global certainty. ˈ

Although my data are drawn from nineteenth-century neurophysiology, the analysis is more generally applicable. Taxonomic uncertainty is common, as Rachel Volberg's study of the species question in biology demonstrates (1983b). She discusses the radically different conceptions that scientists from different disciplines have about what a species is, and she notes a substitution of ideal-type for phenomenological data similar to those discussed here. In Volberg's example, biologists made the substitution as they encountered rare, overlapping, or ephemeral phenomena, and they responded with a search for species exemplars. Yet the basic problem of defining "species" remains technically unsolved.

Similarly, diagnostic puzzles are common, and not simply in medicine. Engineers, for example, often face "buggy" systems that exhibit common symptoms in varying configurations, with individual differences. Many engineering practices, like those described above, may have arisen as an attempt to resolve the overlap of diagnostic, taxonomic, technical, and organizational uncertainties.

Organizational uncertainty is omnipresent in small business endeavors and educational enterprises, professional reform movements, new specialties, and unstable bureaucracies or those with information-processing overloads, to name a few. The development of "safe" commercial products, a focus on small details, and the segmentation of organizations into those dealing with uncertainty and those performing routine tasks are often responses to political uncertainty of the type described here.[5]

Finally, the substitution of theoretical validity for technical certainty, in the face of technically based uncertainty, is common to problem-solving endeavors. The history of psychoanalysis and its critics, for example, shows a continuing debate about the merits of the theory in light of technical uncertainty.

The local contingencies of work are not normally criticized by outsiders, nor open to debate. Thus, when descriptions of them are absent, debates proceed on the basis of published work or lectures. Creating and applying classification systems as well as managing organizational and technical problems (especially of recalcitrant materials), are always part of scientific work. The framework presented here needs to be tested and elaborated in a number of sites, both contemporary and historical, for us to understand more about the process of managing different types of uncertainty in different kinds of organizations.

Much recent work in the sociology and philosophy of science has focused on the production of facts, the treatment of anomalies, and the degree to which theories, once established, are not subject to disconfirmation. Many researchers have noted the persistence of established perspectives or paradigms and the degree to which anomalous information may be ignored if it disconfirms basic assumptions (see, for example, Dewey 1929; Carrier, 1979; Collins and Pinch 1982). Sometimes this is attributed to qualities of the problems themselves; sometimes it is attributed to institutional factors that determine the acceptability of findings. New intermediary variables are sometimes introduced to bridge the hypothesized gap between "internal" and "external."

Despite the wide interest in paradigms and fact production, however, the persistence of perspectives has rarely been analyzed operationally. Such persistence is a characteristic of complex, multiple-site work organization. The analysis presented here posits that the transformation of uncertainty into certainty is one important aspect of the persistence of theories. The transformation is rooted in work organization. This includes local, daily work and larger institutional and political contexts and contingencies, such as sponsorship and the uses of a theory by various audiences.

Theoretical coherence arises as a process. It is the establishment of conventions of production and use, alliances, evaluation criteria, standard operating procedures, and agendas. The continuing power of a perspective in the face of anomalous evidence is an inextricable part of scientific work organization. This is because scientists must work with accountability to both the workplace and the discipline, thus facing many kinds of uncertainty simultaneously.

F O U R

Triangulating Clinical and Basic Research

In the previous chapter, I discussed the conversion of workplace uncertainties into disciplinary certainties through a variety of strategies. One of those strategies was shifting the uncertainties encountered in one domain into another: jettisoning artifacts across the boundaries of work situations. In this chapter, I examine the more general problem of combining data from multiple realms, since it is central both to the localizationist story and to science itself.

The problem here is to analyze the ways in which scientists declare observations from different domains to be evidence of the same phenomenon. Inevitably, as was clear in the previous chapter, the evidentiary sources are mismatched in some way. Phenomena are observed or collected locally, and locales contain unique contingencies. Yet, in order to reach general conclusions, scientists must join evidence drawn from very different realms.

I call this process *triangulation*. Triangulation has two traditional meanings. In geophysical sciences and surveys, it refers to a method of mapping a terrain via multiple measurements taken at different points. Surveyors triangulate to find spots accurately on a territory and to adjust for irregularities in vision peculiar to one site or another. In social sciences and statistics, triangulation has a metaphorically similar meaning: the combination of different measures or viewpoints to make a finding more reliable.

Localizationists triangulated evidence gathered from several types of work, roughly sorted here into clinical and basic realms. These are realms with quite dissimilar standards of evidence, time frames, and work organization. How, and with what consequences, did localizationists join evidence from these dissimilar domains?

The structure of localization theory can be traced back to the work organization of research and clinical practice, particularly via triangulation. The theory's resilience in the face of counterevidence, in particular, is not simply a logical consequence of the structure of scientific theories. We can see it here as a consequence of both uncertainty and triangulation.

Among the outcomes of localizationist research was a functional model of the brain that became widely adopted in medicine and physiology. Localizationist maps, or atlases, reflected the consequences of the triangulation of evidence as practiced by the localizationists. One result of triangulation was the conversion of clinical and basic evidence about individual brains, gathered from local sites, into an ideal form: "*the* brain."

Clinical and Basic Work on Localization

As noted in Chapter 1, many accounts of the history of brain research have presented the work of Ferrier, Jackson, and others as a smooth progression of discoveries and accumulation of facts. Most do not even mention the difficulties of clinical work (but see Cushing 1905, 1910, for exceptions). In general, the picture painted by the history of medicine and physiology has been of steady, unproblematic progress from Jackson's early work on epilepsy, through Ferrier's animal experiments in the 1870's and 1880's and Horsley's neurosurgery of the 1880's and 1890's, to Sherrington's publication of *The Integrative Action of the Nervous System* in 1906. Historians have often characterized this progression as a simple consensus and mutual clarification between clinical and basic fields (such as brain surgery, neurological diagnosis, and animal experimentation).

My investigation into the history of localizationist research forced me to reexamine this picture. I became concerned instead with the extraordinarily complex process of reconciliation between the clean models demanded by scientific audiences and the messy, uncertain facts of everyday worklife. It was clear from the descriptions of daily work conditions as described in hospital records and laboratory notebooks that the integration of clinical and basic results was by no means unproblematic. Localizationists often had to make uneasy coalitions and compromises in combining clinical and basic research. As noted in Chapter 3, each realm faced its own abiding uncertainties, not all of which were resolved either during the 1870–1906 period or later. Furthermore, the purposes and assumptions of the two domains were often contradictory, or at best orthogonal. Because researchers were accountable to both clinical and basic research domains, however, they had to reconcile these approaches to arrive at a general model that would satisfy the demands of both important constituencies (Benton 1978).

Several of the participants in localizationist research were involved in multiple endeavors. For example, Ferrier did physiological experiments and was a practicing neurologist. But since my focus here is on the uses and combination of evidence, I will be using the tasks and lines of work—not individual scientists—as units of analysis.

Triangulations such as those described here, especially those that include clinical as well as basic methods, have always been common in medical science. Among the important unaccounted-for consequences of triangulation are (1) obscuring local uncertainties while emphasizing the "ultimate truth" of a multifaceted model; (2) minimizing individual differences in the service of general findings; and (3) redesigning a theory to meet conflicting requirements from several areas. But there are other, more subtle consequences. The convergence of evidence that appears as abstract in one domain and concrete in another, for example, produces a tricky problem of information management for those seeking to synthesize information (Star 1988a).

The effects of triangulation are particularly apparent in scientific controversies, where evidence for or against one side of a controversy may be adduced without regard to its relationship to other aspects on the same side. The history of localizationist work is a particularly rich topic for the study of this phenomenon, because participants drew heavily on both clinical and basic evidence and there were protracted public arguments about the validity of the theory (Dodds 1877–78; MacCormac 1881; Brown-Séquard 1890a; Swazey 1970).

Cross-Legitimation Between Kinds of Research Evidence

In one of the first localizationist-informed operations, the Queen Square neurosurgeon Victor Horsley collaborated with the neurologist William Gowers to remove a spinal tumor. Gowers performed the neurological localization tests. When Horsley opened the spine where Gowers had predicted, he found no tumor. He had to remove several laminae before he found the tumor—which, had the localization theory been accurate, should have been at a different site. However, as a result of the clinical cure achieved, the operation (like many others) was claimed as a successful instance of localization. Beevor's casebook, 1894 (National Hospital Records), also describes a case in which no tumor was removed but a large amount of bone was removed in the search for it. See also Figure 1, above—the example from Horsley's casebook of the skull progressively opened to cover many different localized sites.

In 1889, American doctors Philip Coombs Knapp and E. H. Bradford had the opposite experience. They reported the death of one of their surgical brain tumor patients after 45 minutes (Knapp and Bradford 1889), but the operation was acclaimed as a success because the tumor *was* located. They note at the beginning of their report the great interest in brain surgery and list 23 cases worldwide of tumor cases located via neurological diagnosis. A similar successful localization, with similar sequelae, was claimed for the first localizationist-informed brain tumor operation, performed by Godlee in 1884 (for more details, see p. 58 above).

What is interesting about these examples is not that clinicians and researchers claimed success for separate domains (sometimes tumors located according to theoretical predictions, sometimes patients cured), but rather that *both* kinds of evidence (clinical success and theoretical prediction) were claimed as support for the theory of localization of brain function. In triangulating, the failures of each realm were discounted in favor of a more general model.

Both the clinical and basic research realms had their own problems with work organization. The uncertainties involved were extensive, as the previous chapter has illustrated. Pathologists lacked comparative data and had difficulty obtaining experimental material. Physiologists had difficulty controlling experimental artifacts and worked in poorly equipped and politically precarious circumstances. Neurologists lacked sophisticated diagnostic systems and faced a bewildering number of symptoms, including the array of epilepsies, some caused by brain tumors and some not. Surgeons faced septic conditions, a lack of good tools, and the opposition of a medical community that thought brain surgery folly (Horsley 1906; Cushing 1910). In addition, both neurologists and surgeons faced uncertainty about whether seizures or dysfunctions were caused by syphilis, tuberculosis, or other diseases for which no reliable diagnostic technology was then available.

More specifically, the several lines of work involved in arguing for localization theory developed clinical and/or basic methods of working that structured the evidence they brought to the argument. The clinical approaches included standard diagnostic taxonomies based on the configuration of symptoms and the administration of neurological tests. The clinical routines of care and observation were based on temporal sequences of events. Doctors performing this research saw disease as localized and removable. The result of this approach was that information tended to be managed on a case-by-case basis. The analysis of physiological mechanisms, comparisons, and interrelationships were minimized. Clinicians emphasized an anatomical perspective: the body seen in terms of structure.

The approaches developed in basic research, by contrast, included decomposition of the brain and nervous system into small, manageable regions and involved what I have called a "blanketing" approach to research. A major research strategy of localizationists was to cover the nervous system by painstakingly identifying and describing discrete parts. This was achieved either by tissue cross-section or by mapping surgical ablations or experimental responses from the cortex. The guiding assumption in basic research was that sooner or later the "whole thing" would get covered. The resulting emphasis was *spatial*. Phenomena tended to be described in terms of space occupied, not time, processes, or sequences of events. Even functional mechanisms were often described spatially as functional regions.

Both the spatial and the anatomical emphases become clear as Jackson (and, later, Ferrier) began to link the order of appearance of symptoms to localization theory. Did epileptic seizures sort into disease categories by region of origin? Doctors eagerly seized on this idea. When Fritsch and Hitzig's localizationist research was published in 1870, it showed, among other things, that convulsions might begin locally and spread. The historian of epilepsy Owsei Temkin discussed the ways in which this idea synthesized clinical and basic work in a significant fashion: "Here indeed was experimental proof for Jackson's clinical observations and pathological inferences. Then Ferrier's experimental work followed and anatomical investigations of the conductive fibres, all of which gave a sound basis for Jackson's contention that localized convulsions indicated localized injuries" (1945: 307). Several strategies were used as researchers and clinicians combined domains of evidence, building on this initial base.

Combining Domains of Evidence

As clinical and basic research realms were combined, the approaches developed in the different lines of work had to be reconciled. This reconciliation took several forms, but two of the most important were: patients as subjects and subjects as patients; and combining political with technical legitimation.

Patients as Subjects and Subjects as Patients

The phrase "experiments made by nature," originally coined by Jackson (1873b), was common in localizationist writings. It represents the view of patients as in vivo experimental "subjects." Scientists from both clinical and basic realms claimed the results of such natural experiments. Surgeons believed that their work validated neurologists' localizations. Physiologists believed that their ablations and electrical applications replicated and stabilized findings from the natural, but uncontrollable, clinical situations. Consider this statement from William MacEwan, a surgeon:

Cerebral surgery has been the means of adding to and confirming the knowledge of brain functions in man, especially of the regions of the cerebral cortex other than motor. . . . In a sense some of these lesions produced in the brain of man may be regarded as experiments carried out by nature with a delicacy, accuracy and refinement which no human experimenter could equal. (1922: 164–65)

The dual role (as clinical treatment and basic research) of surgery in this process is vividly demonstrated by the following description of one of Horsley's operations:

Operation by Mr. Horsley. Patient under morphia and chloroform, parts of the right ascending frontal and parietal convolutions corresponding to the facial centre were removed. (During the operation the surface of the brain was explored with faradic battery and movement of lower jaw, downwards to left obtained and angle of mouth.) (Jackson casebook, 1887, National Hospital Records)

Localizationists were aware of potential weaknesses in combining evidence, but they were limited by work constraints from abandoning either realm or applying more stringent criteria. For example, such "natural experiments" were sometimes criticized by physiologists, but only to the extent that they were taken alone. In triangulating, the "shaky" evidence of clinical "experiments" was combined with physiological results and thus made more robust. No one considered abandoning clinical evidence.

Ferrier, in an article in the localizationist journal *Brain*, described some of the difficulties he experienced in obtaining evidence from the different domains:

I freely admit that in the absence of postmortem confirmation these various facts do not altogether satisfactorily establish a correspondence between the locality of the percussion pain and the cerebral lesion. I have not, however, had an opportunity of postmortem examination in cases which I have carefully examined this way. (1879: 482–83)

Although one ostensible purpose of postmortem examination was to verify the neurological localization of cerebral and other nervous system diseases, this proof became in fact an incidental part of pathological work. Each line of work in effect made the assumption that postmortem findings were consistently correlated with neurological localization. In fact, the lack of topographical sophistication on the part of pathologists and the frequent inability to correlate tumor location with location predicted by neurologists made validation moot. Instead, localizationist theorists simply declared that such correlations were being made. Failures to correlate were frequently ignored.

The original difficulties with these tasks had seemed fairly straightforward to researchers. Ferrier scrawled a quote from François Magendie in one of his notebooks, which reads: "Thanks to the progress of good sense, we prefer the experiment to the most ingenious of 'systems'; the most simple truth appears more beautiful than all the glorious fantasies of the imagination" (1873–1883: December 1874, MS246/4 [my translation]).

Finding these simple truths appeared to be a matter of recreating the one-to-one relationship between area and function that, it was hoped, would be found in the human brain. The logic of experimentation ran thus: delete area, observe dysfunction, then validate existence of functional region. Of course, both physiologists and clinicians quickly found that such a simple approach did not hold, either in applying techniques or in observing results.

Despite the occasional criticism of this nature from both within and outside of the school of thought, localizationist writers, in arguing for the validity of localization of function, usually took evidence in an uncritical fashion from all realms. Physiology was said to correct the uncertainties of clinical work; clinical work was said to provide the validation for physiology. Ferrier, for example, made the following statement in the introduction to his influential 1876 exposition of localization, *The Functions of the Brain*:

Experiments on animals, under conditions selected and varied at the will of the experimenter, are alone capable of furnishing precise data for sound inductions as to the functions of the brain and its various parts; the experiments performed for us by nature, in the form of diseased conditions, being rarely limited, or free from such complications as render analysis and the discovery of cause and effect extremely difficult, and in many cases practically impossible. (p. xiv)

Horsley contrasted surgical data with postmortem data on similar grounds: "Post-mortem records can never teach what the careful study of the living tumours exposed in an operation can demonstrate, since in almost every case the former condition is practically what we may term inoperable" (1906: 411). The neuroanatomist Alfred W. Campbell makes a similar argument for the use of histological data, where physiological and clinical data are seen as imprecise (1905: xi). Yet all three men regularly used clinical, surgical, postmortem pathology, and physiological experiments to argue for localization (see, for example, Ferrier 1878a, 1880, 1881, 1882, 1889, 1890, and especially 1910; Horsley 1891, 1906; Campbell 1905).

Physiologists responded to their lack of institutional security or independent funding by sticking to research that could be justified in clinical terms. Geison (1978) notes that, owing to this dependence, the utilitarian emphasis in medical training also became a "yoke" for physiology. Physiology as taught in the hospital-based medical schools was taught as part of anatomy. "The London hospital schools fostered a utilitarian and correspondingly anatomical conception of physiology. In no way did they provide an insitutional setting conducive to the liberation of physiology from anatomy" (pp. 26–27).

Nor did those training grounds provide any kind of basis for the liberation of physiology from medicine. The triangulation of results from medicine and physiology was important to physiology's continued survival through the turn of the century. Within this situation, physiologists had to develop salable "commodities." Their client was the medical community. Physiologists did struggle to gain a separate institutional base from medicine, as discussed in Chapter 2, but with limited success. This is another important but poorly researched area in the history of physiology. What sorts of questions were supported and which were squelched by its dependence on medicine? At least in the case of localization theory we can see that institutional precariousness was met with a conservative, anatomically oriented approach heavily geared toward clinical validation.

Perhaps because of this institutional situation, physiologists placed great emphasis on situations in which physiological symptoms mirrored disease conditions. In a reverse of the clinical situation described above, where patients were seen as demonstrating physiological hypotheses, physiologists also constructed experiments in which animal subjects were manipulated to reproduce human disease. One of the most famous incidents in localizationist research occurred at the 1881 International Medical Congress in London. This was before the successful localizationist brain tumor operation of 1884.

The German antilocalizationist Goltz and the localizationist Ferrier essentially had a "showdown" at the congress. Goltz brought with him to London several dogs from which he had removed a large portion of the cerebral cortex. His dogs were still mobile and were responsive to commands and stimuli. Goltz believed that these facts refuted localization of motor function in the cortex. He demonstrated the dogs' responsive behavior onstage before the congress audience (MacCormac 1881: 218–37; see also Appendix A of this book). But, following Goltz's demonstration, Ferrier brought a blue-ribbon group of observers with him to his London laboratory, where he kept several monkeys whose brains he had experimentally lesioned. The famous French physician Jean-Martin Charcot was among the visitors. Upon seeing one of the monkeys limping around after having its motor cortex experimentally lesioned, he is said to have exclaimed, "Mais c'est une malade!" (It's a patient!)—likening the monkey to his own hemiplegic patients. (See Thorwald 1959 for a vivid, semi-fictionalized depiction of this scene.)

Charcot's remark was extensively cited in the medical literature, and the demonstration as a whole was widely publicized. Ferrier's experimental subjects were killed. The autopsies were performed by a committee including Gowers and Schafer (Klein, Langley, and Schafer 1883–84; Langley 1883–84a, 1883–84b; Schafer 1883–84). The comparison and matching of symptoms observed both in experimental subjects and in patients provided a crucial double set of evidence for localization. Here was a scientific basis for clinical work and clinical justification for scientific experimentation.

As different types of evidence were triangulated to describe the same phenomenon in a general argument, local contingencies tended to fade. Despite disclaimers about the reliability of various domains, researchers often cited the results of other fields without reference to the uncertainties of work processes. For example, an anatomical atlas by Campbell contains the following passage:

Histologically the area of Broca pertains to the intermediate precentral field; its type of cortex, as displayed by the methods I have employed, does not differ from that situated immediately above, nor from that extending in continuation with it forwards and round. . . . This is of course negative evidence, but it gains in significance when all the data of clinical experience, both the positive and the negative, are considered together with it. (1905: 222)

Campbell was saying that he had failed to find histological differentiation of one presumed functional area of the brain (the famous "speech area"). Yet he did not detail the clinical work that countervailed the negative anatomical evidence, nor did he really criticize it, in that volume. The ultimate effect was that clinical complications were transferred into basic research domains, and, simultaneously, basic research anomalies were transferred into clinical domains. The evidence thus shuffled became intertwined: anomalies were passed between lines of evidence; local uncertainties became buried; and work processes were rendered invisible. Yet the theory gained credibility as many fields added their evidence and helped to manage one another's anomalies.

Political and Technical Alliances

As discussed in Chapter 2, all experimental physiologists had to face the powerful antivivisection movement in the late nineteenth century (French 1975). Localizationists, like many other physiological researchers, combined the validation of their theories with the political question of whether any vivisectionist research was legitimate. Localizationists often answered the political criticisms with an appeal to the clinical importance of the research. Any opponent of vivisection thus became converted, in localizationist rhetoric, into an opponent of the theory.

An ongoing alliance against a common enemy had been forged between British physiologists and the medical profession, with localization research as an important part of it (French 1975: 203). Events subsequent to the Ferrier-Goltz showdown further cemented the political/technical alliance for localizationism. Ferrier was arrested and tried under the 1876 Cruelty to Animals Act on charges of having performed surgery on his monkeys without a license. Although, as detailed in Chapter 2, Ferrier was acquitted, his trial cemented in the public mind the links between vivisection, physiology as a legitimate research enterprise, and localization theory.

Crichton-Browne's 1884 letter to the London *Times* following the first localizationist brain operation (quoted above, p. 81) illustrates the combination of clinical, political, and technical validity. It underscores the complex politics of interchange between clinical and basic evidence. The message was clear: animal life versus human life was directly at stake in the localizationist arena. If one opposes animal experimentation, one sacrifices human life.

Because localization was at first heavily disputed even within the provivisectionist scientific community, some triangulation took place in response to antilocalizationist attacks (Panizza 1887; Brown-Séquard 1890a, 1890b). On the one hand, Ferrier and others assembled evidence from all lines of work to counter diffusionist arguments and make cases. On the other hand, much triangulation was "internal" to the localizationist school of thought in the sense that anomalies encountered in clinical or physiological research were answered by evidence from other localizationist domains. External debates and internal syntheses thus blended into one another in the pages of journals, in books, and in demonstrations (Ferrier 1876: 233–35).

Triangulation Strategies: General Issues in the Philosophy of Medicine

What can we say in a general way about triangulation strategies from this analysis of clinical and basic work organization? What implications does it have for a theory of information, science, and work organization?

If an argument or result must draw on several lines of work, it must in some sense account for the commitments and points of view developed by each. For localizationists, the impact of combining evidence from the different realms in which they worked was enormous.

In the social and biological sciences, triangulation usually refers to a methodological tool for improving validity or reliability. Validity means better information about events occurring at a site. Reliability refers to whether those events can be reproduced.

Thus triangulation has two meanings: it can refer to the use of the *same* method employed repeatedly by independent researchers to describe the same object, or it can refer to the use of *different* methods, also taken independently, to describe the same object. The first use is meant to correct for local or idiosyncratic misapplications of a technique by presuming that everyone will not make the same local mistakes in application. It does not, however, account for biases inherent in the tool itself. It compares users, not tools.

The second use, which is much more powerful, applies multiple methods to describe the same object. Because it implicitly compares measures as well as users, the results it yields are more robust. The assumption behind this type of triangulation is that the failings or biases of one method will be corrected for by the use of another. For instance, one might use survey research, interviews, and demographic data to triangulate on the same social phenomenon. By examining convergence and divergence of results, it is theoretically possible to ensure more robust results (Campbell and Fiske 1959; Wimsatt 1981).

There is an aspect of this second kind of triangulation that has been poorly understood on a practical basis by medical historians, philosophers, and medical researchers. This is the synthetic sense. When researchers draw on evidence from different realms to describe the same phenomenon, they are triangulating with different measures; they are trying to eliminate or correct for the biases inherent in a single point of view.

The methodological problem is not a new one. William Whewell's 1847 framing of the problem of "consilience of inductions" called for a method of combining evidence to achieve truth. His consilience process had three satisfying criteria: that independent processes arrive at the same hypothesis; that the new hypothesis be able to predict unexpected new facts; and that it have a "tendency to simplicity and harmony." That is, the new hypothesis should parsimoniously explain the new phenomena without a great deal of ad hoc revision (Whewell 1967 [1847]; Laudan 1981).

From Whewell on, triangulation as a tool for increasing robustness has theoretically rested on the independence of combined measures, in order not to produce a "folie à deux" (or à any number) situation. But as Donald Campbell and D. W. Fiske discuss in their classic article, independence of measures is a continuum, not an either/or proposition. To the extent that measures are independent, convergence measures validity; to the extent that they are not, convergence measures reliability. In the case where multiple, semi-independent measures are being adduced to argue for the same phenomenon, there is a real lack of clarity about whether reliability or validity is being measured. (See also Lasagna 1972 for a comparable example of this confusion in measuring the efficacy of pharmaceutical drug trials.)

Yet traditional prescriptive discussions of triangulation have excluded analysis of the bases on which evidence is developed in the different realms. I refer here to differences in epistemology: different presentational constraints, conventions and standards for significance of findings, historical and institutional emphases, and the political acceptability of different ways of knowing things. All discussions of triangulation to date have excluded the structural conditions of work, daily work contingencies, histories and traditions of lines of work, and the processes of triangulating evidence, including attributing certainty to other fields.

These omissions can be traced to a general lack of emphasis among most philosophers on contextual analyses of reasoning, a lack of emphasis among sociologists on the work organization and institutional bases of scientific knowledge, and a lack of emphasis among medical historians on the changing nature and development of social systems of argument and work organization. Although this has recently begun to change, there has been little direct research that—in a thoroughly empirical way—examines the conditions and consequences of combining evidence.

Because of these omissions, the possibility of interlocking biases, of buried uncertainties, and of what Wimsatt (1981) calls "bias amplification" and "pseudorobustness" has been neglected; more important, the common-sense view in science that more agreeing views make more robust findings has not been looked at empirically in light of institutional and daily work contingencies. Oskar Morgenstern's *On the Accuracy of Economic Observations* (1963) provides an elegant critique of this problem from the point of view of data collection and statistics.

Some discussion of the importance of philosophical and epistemological differences as based on practice between clinical and basic approaches has appeared in the philosophy of medicine literature. Patrick Heelan (1977) makes a convincing argument that the exigencies of work and available technology form the context for joining clinical and basic research and frame its biases. He says that clinical science is composed of concrete, practical knowledge, which then turns to general principles to explain events. It does not proceed on the basis of elaborating general systems. "In clinical science, the immediacy of knowledge is not basic science, but typically a skillfully designed instrument based on good basic science and good technological principles of design. . . . Clinical science is basic science incorporated nonobjectively" (p. 30).

King (1982) has also lucidly described the relationship between diagnostic taxonomies, nosology (medical taxonomy), and symptoms. He, too, ties it to the exigencies of work in particular specialties, and he says that specialists elaborate taxonomies and make them increasingly precise. This certainly was the case in the localizationist research setting, since increased knowledge of fine-grained taxonomies can influence therapeutic choice. In the long run, however, clinicians will only use categories that prove clinically useful. "For the clinician, 'use' refers to the value in promoting cure. In research, however, 'use' might mean the value in promoting understanding" (p. 103).

It is precisely the flow of understandings that King describes, and the pragmatic requirements of the occasions to which he refers, that this chapter charts. The requirements are the everyday needs faced by workers in identifying and sorting various clinical and physiological phenomena. Geison (1977) has provided an excellent description of such practical organizational differences in clinical and basic physiological work. For localizationists, these buried uncertainties and interlocking contingencies were a central part of the organization of work of researching brain function.

The uncertainties of clinical work have received attention elsewhere, particularly in the philosophy of medicine and in medical technology. Strauss et al. (1985), for example, discuss many of the uncertainties in clinical medicine and the complexity of "articulating" the various kinds of work entwined in the hospital. This uncertainty comes to the fore in the attempted development of computer-based "expert systems," which try to recapitulate, automate, or rationalize "clinical judgment" (Shortliffe 1976). Edmond Murphy's excellent discussions of clinical classification systems (1977, 1982; see also Meehl 1977); Stephen Toulmin's work on physicians' reasoning (1976); Harry Marks's excellent review of randomized clinical trials (1984); and an extensive literature in medical sociology (such as Becker et al. 1961; Freidson 1968, 1970b) all indicate that there are large gaps between the clinician's work and experience and the systems of basic science that attempt to incorporate clinical findings. Trevor Pinch (1980) provides a sociological analysis of the similar problem of combining applied and theoretical work in physics.

In the presence of these gaps, the triangulation of clinical and basic results is often ad hoc or uneven, contributing to confounded debates and findings whose significance may be difficult to assess. An analysis of the work organization is needed to understand the relationship between different commitment structures and the processes of triangulation described here. In the next section I analyze some of the general characteristics of clinical and basic work and the consequences of their combination.

Building the Brain with Both Clinical and Basic Perspectives

The different views that informed localizationist clinical and basic research resulted, in the former case, in a view of disease as localized and removable and, in the latter case, in a spatial approach to physiological problems. But in a more general sense, there were important differences between clinical and basic work that informed the triangulation process. Imagine a braid composed of heterogeneous elements: how does the braiding proceed smoothly?

The very different commitment structures of the clinical and basic realms were transformed by the triangulation of evidence into a single harmonious realm. Physiologists relied on clinical evidence to supplement their anomalous, uncertain, or perhaps politically unsavory (to antivivisectionists) results. When the different approaches and limitations outlined above were combined to argue for localization, the following consequences for localization theory ensued.

1. The unit of analysis was plastic. Clinical work was primarily geared toward individual problems and their solution; basic research was geared toward aggregates or statistical units. The result of triangulating these differences was that case evidence became evidence for analytic principles in physiology, and vice versa. Thus the actual unit of analysis for the theory as a whole became unclear, and it expanded or shrank to fit the boundaries of the immediate problem under discussion. Another result here was a minimizing of individual differences. In sum: individual cases as unit (clinical) + aggregate approaches (basic) = unclear unit of analysis, with plastic boundaries.

2. The direction of abstraction yielded an ideal type. In the words of the medical sociologist Eliot Freidson, "The practicing physician may use general principles to deal with concrete problems; the scientist typically investigates concrete phenomena in order to test, elaborate, or arrive at general principles" (1970b: 163). The use and direc-

tion of abstraction was different in the two enterprises. This meant that evidence traveling in two directions, in a metaphorical sense, was combined. The result was a slippery, unfalsifiable base of evidence. This stemmed from the lack of either an empirical base or rigorous logical requirements that simple abstraction or exemplification would require. (Griesemer and Wade 1988 discuss some of the properties of abstraction and causality that inform this analysis.) In sum: direction of abstraction from concrete → abstract (clinical) + direction of abstraction from abstract → concrete (basic) = ideal type.

3. Different temporal orientations led to a lack of developmental emphasis. Clinical work was oriented toward immediate results: the patient must be cured now, before the results of the basic research may be fully incorporated. (Even in the hospitals for the chronically ill, such as Queen Square, there was an urgency to treating patients and resolving cases.) Basic research, on the other hand, was geared toward posing and solving problems that would be a thorough description of the general situation. The time horizon was remote for any individual case. The result of this combination was a lack of emphasis on any temporal concerns beyond those observable in the short-term clinical site (such as the march of symptoms described by Jackson 1873a, 1931). In sum: short temporal orientation (clinical) + long temporal orientation (basic) = atemporality and a lack of developmental approaches.

4. A different orientation toward anomalies supported the shifting of anomalous evidence between realms. Anomalies were interruptions to the routine performance of work, pieces of information or research that did not fit expected findings. They included accidents, mistakes, artifacts, and discoveries (Star and Gerson 1987). Clinical anomalies were complications: those events that inhibited or prohibited the administration of therapies, diagnostic procedures, or patient responses to therapies. Their management consisted primarily in insulating and eradicating the case-level mistake or accident. Basic research anomalies, by contrast, were interruptions to a chain of inference or experimental procedures. They thus prohibited smooth progress to a set of generalized results. Their management consisted primarily in determining the impact of the anomaly on the chain of inference: was it significant, acceptable, or controllable? Where clin-

ical science saw complications that may threaten patients, basic research saw artifacts that may impeach the validity of findings if not handled correctly. The result of combining evidence with these very different approaches to anomalies was the sort of shuffle of misfitted evidence between domains described above and in Chapter 3. In sum: orientation toward anomalies as complications (clinical) + orientation toward anomalies as theoretical contingencies (basic) = discarding anomalies from both realms into the other; invisibility of anomalous evidence.

5. Physiological investigations were described anatomically. Anatomical/surgical evidence from individual cases was added to the results of physiological investigation and used to frame physiological problems as spatial problems of location. The atemporality that was a result of combining different time frames, the spatial emphasis of research, and the lack of developmental emphasis combined to substitute anatomy for physiology.

6. Diagnostic taxonomies became basic research taxonomies, and vice-versa. Physiological researchers adopted the strategy of trying to match or produce disease locations in their subjects; clinicians wrote up cases using basic research taxonomies. A *modular* theory was thus created, whose components could be "plugged in" or worked on in interchangeable pieces without violating either kind of taxonomy. Many of the clinical and basic results on localization were reported as small, modular parts of a larger theory. Cases were reported as instantiating one particular functional area of the brain; experiments that mapped discrete brain areas were emphasized (Beevor and Horsley 1890, 1894; Hobson 1882; Rabagliati 1878a, 1878b).[1]

To summarize: neurologists and pathologists, through their daily work organization, held the individual as a robust unit of analysis. They analyzed problems in terms of individuals or cases. Physiologists, on the other hand, took universal structure as their unit of analysis. Surgeons had two types of analysis, depending on whether they were searching for anatomical structures or for ways to block tumor growth, bleeding, or infection. For the most part, they had a practical need to operate quickly and accurately, to make incisions and find tumors as predicted by the neurologists. This quickness was prompted by the increased risk of infection the longer a wound stayed open. Records indicate that Horsley could remove a brain tumor, including making the incision through the skull, in 15 minutes (Jones 1946)! Thus they did not have the time, resources or methods to analyze the individuality of brain structures.

In physiology, the need to find universal structures led to an attempt to replicate, in animals, disease conditions existing in humans. But the match was not between Mrs. Jones's left temporal brain tumor and Edna the monkey's laboratory-produced lesion. Instead, physiologists tried to reproduce situations that would mirror *any* brain tumor so located. The reproduction of disease was directed toward general principles, not specific laboratory settings. The physiologists' mandate was to validate general taxonomies, not individual cases. Thus, at the same time that the individual become the robust unit of analysis in two disciplines, individual differences were ignored by other fields seeking to validate their work. Individual case boundaries were combined with an absence of analysis of individual differences.

These consequences reflect the conflicting demands of the clinical and basic realms: different time horizons, methods of managing anomalies, generalizations, and the other aspects of work organization discussed here. One concrete product of localizationist work that incorporated these emphases and was used in both clinical and basic work was functional maps or atlases of the brain. These atlases were in part road maps meant for clinicans faced with seizures and symptoms of tumors, a guide to "localizing signs"; they were also ideal typologies of the functions of the brain, nonempirical arguments for localization of function.

This somewhat contradictory situation created the need for universal maps that would be applicable in individual cases. These maps had to incorporate function (the problem of neurologists and physiologists) with structure (the problem of surgeons and pathologists) in an exposition usable by working doctors. Localization theory was developed in response to this multiple set of needs by applying both structure and function simultaneously.

Localizationist maps were designed to be tools that would accommodate the needs and standards of both clinicians and basic researchers. But they did not address individual differences, and they glossed lightly over interspecies differences. Such maps became an important source of legitimation for localization theory. They were widely adopted in medical texts of all kinds, and indeed they form the basis of our modern picture of the brain. These maps also appear as simple facts, testaments to certainty and consensus arising from a complex braiding of uncertainty and compromise (see, for example, the maps in Ferrier 1876 and Gowers 1885).

Summary

Understanding the ways in which researchers combine evidence from clinical and basic domains is critical for the history of medicine because of the extensive reliance on both clinical and basic research in the past and the present. The history of medicine as a field has undergone many changes in the 1970's and 1980's, and there is a much greater desire to understand both the social/political contexts of research and clinical care and the technical medical details that concern researchers and clinicians. Many gaps remain, however. One important gap is the lack of analysis of clinical and basic work—not as lists of great discoveries or great physicians, but as organized technical activities historically situated. Understanding the nature of the work organization that produces clinical and basic results, and the differences between them, is a critical first step to understanding the consequences of triangulation and the significance and degree of convergent results.

Perhaps a more fundamental result of this analysis goes beyond the history of medicine and its recording of clinical and basic combinations or convergences. I began this chapter with the problem posed as follows: under what conditions do scientists declare observations from different domains to be evidence of the same phenomenon? That is, how do they reconcile divergent criteria of evaluation for results that arise from differences in work organization in different domains?

In Chapters 3 and 4 I have detailed the strategies by which localizationist researchers created certainty and closure for their theory. These strategies speak to an important aspect of scientific knowledge: its *distributed* nature. At no one point in time or space can a piece of scientific evidence, or even the work of one scientist, be said to represent a theory in its entirety. Theories are distributed over multiple sites and over long periods of time. No central authority evolves, adjudicates, or disseminates theories.

This has some important implications for our understanding of the growth of scientific knowledge. First, the bits and pieces collectively assembled to produce scientific knowledge are *heterogeneous* (Law 1987). That is, because there is no central authority or distribution system, each locality and each work site develops local approaches, evaluation criteria, and local knowledge about phenomena. When these are combined, it is as heterogeneous parts; the whole is an ever-evolving, decentralized system.[2]

Perspectives are incomplete at any one point, an observation that has had fundamental importance in mathematics and physics. Yet social scientists have been slow to mine the implications of this observation, as Bentley (1926) observed many years ago. The point is simple, yet bears repeating: in the absence of a central authority, local findings will vary with local conditions. The transformations that knowledge undergoes as it is joined across sites and is transformed to certainty at larger scales of organization represent virtually unknown territory. No purely logical analysis of the structure of a scientific theory can capture these transformations, because they are local to the experience of investigators at different sites. Those investigators follow no particular logical dictums in coping with the exigencies of their situations; they must handle patients with seizures and infections, recalcitrant monkeys, political movements, and stubborn colleagues.

Latour (1988) has spoken of "equivalence negotiations" as being the stuff of scientific knowledge and power: those negotiations that take place about what evidence can be joined from where in creating knowledge. This chapter has been a study in equivalence negotiations, their complexity and often unforeseen consequences. Many questions remain to be answered in this area. A more thorough analysis of the conventional approaches developed in both clinical and basic research realms is needed to flesh out the picture presented here, especially as these approaches changed from era to era and from place to place.

Another rich field for investigation would be analysis of the possible impacts of hierarchies of credibility (Becker 1967) on different fields. That is, people see certain disciplines, individuals, and institutions as more prestigious or credible in different times and places. The word of a physician automatically carries more weight (with most people) than that of a derelict, regardless of the logical truth values of their statements. The analysis of triangulation should include an understanding of the different weighting of evidence from differently credible domains.[3]

In the next chapter, I analyze another aspect of distributed knowledge: debate. Here it is not the relatively peaceful reconciliation of widely different standards at stake, but a bitter dispute about localization theory.

FIVE

The Debate About Cerebral Localization

Localizationism was not universally accepted from the beginning of the endeavor. In fact, as noted in the previous chapter, one major impetus for triangulation of evidence was that localizationists were called upon from early days to defend their theories to unfriendly audiences. By culling evidence from different spheres, they could meet criticism with adequate counterpoints. The debate about localization was most fierce from the early 1870's to the mid-1890's, the period reviewed in this chapter. But, in fact, the debate continued after this, and indeed it continues today.

The purpose of this chapter is not simply to demonstrate that there was opposition to localization, but also to examine the ways in which, in Georg Simmel's words (1903–4), conflict socializes its participants. A scholarly debate is not simply an exchange of opinions. It is a series of publications, demonstrations, and commitments to lines of action—none of which are easily retracted or quickly responded to. The more widespread and multifaceted the issues in the debate, the more subtly entrenched the assumptions of both sides become. Debates in this way obscure as well as illuminate.

Several kinds of argument were entangled in the cerebral localization debate in the nineteenth century. These included questions about whether cerebral localization existed at all, or whether the brain could be divided into functional areas. These in turn blended into questions about the extent of localization. Some critics felt that cerebral localization probably existed, but to what extent? Did it exist in both animals and humans? If only in animals, which ones? In the cerebral hemispheres as well as the lower brain centers, or the spinal cord? If not, where did the phenomenon stop, and why? Was localized function as specific as one region per function? Or could it be two regions, one function? Several regions, one function? If the latter were the case, could we then speak of functions being duplicated or distributed over the brain? And finally, did localization of function in the brain imply a similar kind of organization throughout the rest of the nervous system?

These questions were by no means clearly distinguished either by critics or by proponents. In addition, questions about causality and consequences of localization of function were included in the controversy. Critics and proponents alike questioned the cause of the phenomena observed in localization experiments and clinical data. Were the phenomena evolutionary, anatomical, or socially derived? Were they caused by the distribution of different kinds of cells throughout the brain (Campbell 1905) or by functional differentiation at the endpoint of nerve pathways? Did events and abilities become located in the brain via chemicals, associations, or electrical storage?

The uses of localization were also in question. Clinicians wondered whether theories of localization of function could be used to diagnose diseases of the nervous system. Philosophers hoped that it might explain the nature of the mind and perhaps resolve some of the oldest philosophical questions about the relationship between brain and mind. Others questioned whether localization of function was a good way to view human beings at all. Did it have potentially good or bad consequences for the philosophy of human nature? Did it imply determinism and lack of free will, as William James and others seemed to imply? Was even doing the research itself a good or a bad thing?

Scientists often intermingled these several types of debate. Simultaneous arguments proceeded, for example, about whether localization existed at all, if it existed only in animals, whether duplication of functions occurred, and, if so, did it mean that localization did not exist after all? All of these arguments proliferated—in the medical and scientific press, in medical congresses and demonstrations, and in professional associations.

Meanwhile, localization-based practices were rapidly established in hospitals, medical education institutions, and physiological laboratories. Patients and the public were being educated (through the popular press and through doctors) about its merits and meanings. Several things derived from this proliferation during the course of the debate. First, the subdebates became conflated. Participants often raised one kind of issue and were answered with another. They would give an example from one domain of evidence and receive a counter-example from another, as with the triangulation of evidence discussed in Chapter 4. Second, as anomalies arose in the course of research and daily work, researchers would find them explained in published de-nunciations of antilocalizationists, then rebutted by localizationist writings. Thus, daily work concerns were addressed in a larger sphere and against a common enemy. Third, within a given line of work, arguments were often confounded. That is, participants talked past one another, answering in terms that not only did not address the original questions but changed their questions by substituting differ-ent concerns.

Debates are often conceived of as simply verbal or written inter-changes. But in any debate, including scientific ones, the weaponry is only partly linguistic. Demonstrations, solutions to technical prob-lems, successful operations, lobbying, voting, and funding were all invoked or used as debating strategies (see Latour 1988 for a discus-sion of a similar phenomenon in Pasteur's work).

The institutional contexts, everyday work, and disciplinary lines of work described thus far have alternately been figure and ground for one another. The antilocalizationist debate adds a third layer to this analysis. Debating with diffusionists affected the daily work situation by providing arguments for dismissing or packaging up many kinds of anomaly encountered in the laboratories and clinics. The debate also affected the institutional context of localizationism by defining a public in-group united against a common enemy.

As noted above, the debaters represented a wide range of interests and lines of work: neurology, surgery, pathology, physiology, hos-pital administration, philosophy, journalism, antivivisection, and pa-tients and their families. These groups adopted different and overlap-ping debating positions.

During the period considered here, these multiple positions strengthened one another in complex ways. Like the strands of a braid, they became stronger in conjunction than any one argument alone. As with triangulation, such conjunctions become quite complex and persistent. Although the participants almost never addressed either the *logic of conjunction* of the arguments or the connections between their work and their debating positions, they drew from one another's positions and from the circumstances of their daily work to weave a pattern of argument and proof that is extraordinarily dense. The situation was described by Horsley's biographer, Paget:

> After 1875, the output of work, in this and other countries, became so great that no man can describe it. The main lines of it are clear enough. One was the application of the facts of cerebral localization to the study of injuries and diseases of the brain, with special reference to cases of "Jacksonian epilepsy." Another was the advancement of the surgery of the brain. Another was the incessant criticising and interpreting and adjusting of all new facts and theories as they came to hand. Another was the modern study of the deeper parts of the brain, and of the spinal cord. Along these and other lines, all of them crossing and recrossing, legions of men were at work. (1919: 94)

"Winning" the localization debate was thus a complicated progression of events. Its logic and progress are not found in the rules of a game, but rather in an analysis of the kinds of work entangled in its momentum. From 1870 to the mid-1890's, concepts of the localization of brain function and the resulting picture of the brain/mind relationship became increasingly tied to a number of going concerns in medicine, physiology, and psychology (Walker 1957), as discussed in Chapter 2.

Debating, then, is like Simmel's analysis of conflict (1903–4). Debates are not just words; they carry their own organizational weight. Conflict is itself socializing, in that participation in conflict reflects and develops commitments to certain paths of action. After a long period of time, the very density and durability of the debate forms a structure of its own. Battle lines are drawn, and the topics of debate provide a wellspring of problems for research and publication. Career directions are defined with reference to the debate.

Critics of Localization Theory: The Diffusionists

Criticism of localization was unorganized, albeit vehement and sustained. Information on the opponents of localization is sparse. Furthermore, critics' positions were not monolithic. Diffusionists attacked the theory of localization of function on several different grounds, developing and drawing on alternative theories of nervous function. This chapter focuses primarily on their interactions with the group at Queen Square and on the dynamics of the debate.

Who were the diffusionists? Among the most vocal and prominent was Charles-Edouard Brown-Séquard, a Mauritian physiologist-physician who worked in France, England, Mauritius, and the United States. He was briefly a student of Jackson's, and some of their common concerns are reflected in analyses of the effects of tumors and lesions in producing seizures. In 1878 he succeeded Claude Bernard as the chair of medicine at the Collège de France. In the course of his famous and pioneering research on epilepsy, Brown-Séquard, like Jackson, developed a theory of "action at a distance" and "remote effects" to explain the relationship between lesions and dysfunctions. He believed that lesions could exert a distant influence anywhere in the nervous system and that this influence could either inhibit or excite function. He named these two counterbalanced forces in the body "inhibition" and "dynamogenesis." Unlike Jackson, however, Brown-Séquard believed that it was the influence of these organism-wide forces, and not of discrete regions of the brain with individual functions, that caused seizures and other symptoms. Brown-Séquard used these concepts to explain the same phenomena that Ferrier, Jackson, and Horsley thought to be localized in the cerebral cortex. Brown-Séquard and the group at Queen Square engaged in a bitter debate about localization that lasted for a number of years (see, for example, Brown-Séquard 1873a, 1873b, 1879; Olmsted 1946; Role 1977).

Friedrich Goltz, another prominent antilocalizationist, was a German physiologist who was primarily interested in nervous inhibition and related phenomena. His methods were similar to those of the localizationists. Like them, he produced lesions in animal cortexes and observed the effects. He performed a number of experiments in which he removed the cortex of the animal and then observed the effects of near-total decortication. Goltz attempted to refute localizationism by showing that animals without large parts of their cerebral cortex were still able to perform many functions thought to be localized there. When he removed the areas localizationists supposed responsible for motor movements, for instance, his animals still walked, ate, and responded to contact. Goltz held that this indicated the absence of discrete sensory-motor areas (Goltz 1881; see also Appendix A).

Two other critics indicative of the diverse opposition to localizationism were Mario Panizza and William James. Panizza was an Italian physiologist who criticized the idea of functional centers and what he saw as methodological and philosophical problems in localizationist theory. He maintained that localizationism was in a sense a "category error": it could not be directly proved or disproved by direct evidence, because there was no basis for causality in the way localizationists approached the issue.[1] That is, he held that simultaneously observing a deleted or damaged region and some sort of dysfunction proved nothing about causal connections between the two. Like Brown-Séquard, he pointed out that there can be many reasons to smile or kick that do not require the existence of a "smile center" or "kick center." He saw the nervous system as composed of complex, labile, redundant forces that were interactive.

Like the Pragmatist philosophers who criticized the concept of reflex in psychology, Panizza argued that sensations could not be truly localized. Such a model would require that sensation enter at one place and come out at another, meanwhile "stopping" somewhere to be processed by a (nonexistent) overseeing function (for example, Bentley 1975b; Dewey 1981 [1896]). Panizza's model of the nervous system (1887) was more temporally fluid than the localizationists' (see also Appendix B). That is, he saw nervous or behavioral responses as not necessarily predicated on event A directly precipitating event B; instead, a complex interactive response could include delays, repetition, and culmination.

Panizza's research and criticism was virtually ignored by English physiologists, although his book went into two editions in Italy. I found only one review of his work in the English-language press (Rabagliati 1882). By contrast, Italian localizationists such as Luciani and Tamburini were heavily cited in the English-language medical literature.

William James, the American philosopher and psychologist, provided a lively critique of many aspects of the work of the localizationists in his *Principles of Psychology* (1890). James, like Panizza, saw problems with the conceptual foundations of strict localizationism, especially as it conceived of complex behaviors. James believed that all behavior was contextual and that it acquired meaning only in light of goals and social interactions. Thus, if functional control of behavior was rooted in anatomy or in some static location, one would encounter serious epistemological problems. How could one site determine many behaviors? What mechanisms of adaptation could there be? Much of reflex psychology and physiology as well as localizationist philosophy seemed to James to be idealist. That is, they relied on nonempirical systems of understanding that could not be verified by direct experience. Strictly speaking, however, James was not a diffusionist; he also agreed (in what seems to me a contradictory way) with many of the localizationists' positions, especially about sensory and motor localization (see his 1890: vol. 1, pp. 30–43).

He succinctly stated the nature of much diffusionist criticism in the following passage:

In presence of such discord as that between [localizationist] Munk and his opponents one must carefully note how differently significant is *loss*, from *preservation*, of a function after an operation on the brain. The *loss* of a function does not necessarily show that it *is* dependent on the part cut out; but its *preservation* does show that it is *not* dependent; and this is true though the loss should be observed ninety-nine times and the preservation only once in a hundred similar excisions. (1890: vol. 1, p. 43)

James relied on the arguments of Goltz and Brown-Séquard to demonstrate the philosophical and psychological complexity of the subject. He also reproduced several of the localizationists' diagrams of the brain's functions, including those of Ferrier, Munk, and Luciani.

General Form of the Debate

The debate about localizationism at first proceeded slowly, partly because of the structural position of localizationist experimenters within the medical reform movement and specialty hospitals. Between 1870 and 1873, localizationist research burgeoned in England and on the continent. After Ferrier's research (following the lead of Fritsch and Hitzig) was published in 1873, the approach began to draw more serious criticism. However, by the time most of the detailed criticism appeared, localizationists had already begun to establish their program of research and clinical care. Localization experiments were

proliferating. Diffusionists were at a disadvantage both organizationally and in the timing of their critiques.

The general flow of the debate was as follows. The localizationists
published the results of brain-mapping experiments or case studies
and claimed this as evidence for area-specific functions originating in
the brain. This evidence was then attacked by diffusionists (such as
Brown-Séquard in 1879) or by other localizationists who disagreed
about method or the precise location of functional regions. These attacks presented different hypotheses about the source of specific functions (Knapp and Bradford 1889), whether the source could indeed
be considered unique, and the validity of the methods used to detect
them. As time went on, the issues raised by diffusionists were often
incorporated into localizationist models yet explained within the analytic framework of localization.[2]

Brown-Séquard's challenges, as well as those of Panizza and Goltz
(see Appendixes), were not successful in the sense of getting the localizationists to change research direction or abandon their enterprises. Yet they had an important effect on the content of localization
theory. This effect has gone virtually unnoticed by historians of neurophysiology, perhaps because it seems counterintuitive that an opposing point of view should play such an important role in the positive development of a theory.

The criticisms raised by diffusionists *were* addressed by localizationists. Sometimes they were assimilated, sometimes directly rebutted, and sometimes diplomatically put on the sidelines or insulated
from serious discussion. But in the process of meeting the criticisms,
localizationists developed a powerful technology for arguing and
thereby greatly strengthened their position.

Arguments are not usually thought of as technologies. Yet they
perform many of the same information-handling functions as scientific instruments. As localizationists argued with diffusionists, they
confronted anomalies and irregularities in the data and argued about
the significance of phenomena. As this became routine, pools of argument developed with which localizationists could handle classes of
anomaly. Inconstant relations between area and function, for example, became a well-argued point. Instead of being a persistent uncertainty in daily work, it was transformed into a point of doctrine for

localizationists. They developed a repertoire of answers to explain problems with inconstant relations. This repertoire was created in large part as a result of debate. (Some of these answers are analyzed in Chapter 7, since they form an important part of the persistence of localization theory through the modern period.)

In general, localizationists posited several kinds of answers to diffusionist criticism about the failures of localization predictions. These were principally:

1. Redundancy of function. The organism could still function with one "*x* center" impaired because in fact there are multiple centers for this function in the brain. For example, there would be not just one "speech center" but many, scattered over different parts of the cortex.

2. Recovery of function. Because more than one area can be responsible for a function, some areas can act as a sort of backup for damaged regions.

3. Methodological inadequacy. The anomalies are due to failures in measurement technology. This technology is currently inadequate for conclusive demonstration of functional regions, but in the future technologies will bear out the theory.

Thus, in addition to daily work and institutional concerns, the shape of localization theory was developed through conflict with its opponents. In its simplest form, this book could be read as arguing that localizationists "won" a scientific debate because they controlled more resources and linked their arguments to successful enterprises. But winning the debate is only one part of the analysis of the development of the perspective. The actual content of the final theory was shaped in a far more dialectical fashion. Furthermore, its legacy persists in the form of those assumptions embedded in the debate and in the practices—a complex clotting of logic and work.

Stylistic Conflicts

Scientific debates, like formal forensics or legislative battles, consist of far more than point-for-point logic. The reasons for allegiance to one side or another vary, from tacit to explicit and from the traditionally logical to a range of other reasons including political alliance. When scientists from organizations with sharply differing approaches or styles disagree about results, they are often unable to communicate, and they end up speaking past one another's logics. They are committed to approaching problems in certain ways. These overall approaches to the world are rooted in "ultimate questions" about nature. Styles may vary along several dimensions, including the atomistic-holistic—that is, from the atomistic (nature is composed of discrete particles, added together to form a whole) to the systemic (nature is an inviolable whole, and things operate together to form a unity, also called gestalt).

The localizationists were atomistic in style; diffusionists were systemic. Thus the debate about localization of function in the brain is, among other things, a debate between incompatible styles about the nature of nature. (There were also arguments *within* the localizationist camp about the extent or location of specific areas; as noted in Chapter 3, these conflicts also served to strengthen the localizationist position.)

Such conflict densely marks the history of biology: for example, in the battle between Santiago Ramon y Cajal and Camillo Golgi about whether nerves are continuous or discrete; in reproductive biology, the debate about whether reproductive cells reproduce in particulate or systemic fashion (Clarke 1985); and in biology, the conflict between naturalists and experimenters (Rainger, Benson, and Maienschein 1988).

The sociology and history of science have paid relatively little attention to the formal properties of scientific debates, although there have been some excellent case studies. These include Martin Rudwick's important case study of a controversy in nineteenth-century geology (1985).

A scientific problem becomes a debate when workers disagree about what needs to be done next. Negotiations will continue if participants refuse to change bargaining positions. The scope of these debates can be large or small; they may be prolonged or short-lived. Debates that occur across several lines of work involve alliances as well as arguments. That is, multiple traditions and ways of working are at stake in the debate about what necessary next steps can in fact solve the problem. Debates thus become relatively stable foci for work and conflict. Stylistic conflicts, because they are irreconcilable, may actually help stabilize the arena. Goltz, for example, complained of being transformed into the symbolic "loyal opposition" in the localizationist-diffusionist debate, despite certain agreements with the localizationists:

> In the meantime I went along my own way. Even if I was convinced that the assumption of small circumscribed centers did not correspond with the facts, that did not mean that the idea of Flourens, that the substance of the brain was equivalent everywhere, was correct. I tried to find out what consequences the amputation of single lobes of the brain had, and found that the destruction of the anterior lobes led to entirely different disturbances from the destruction of the occipital lobes. In this direction, too, I could rectify Flourens' ideas. Instead of thanking me, the proponents of cerebral centers have accused me of fleeing from the colors. It should be my business to deny any localization. If I now admit a certain localization, I denounce my former sins, so I was told. (1950 [1888]: 129–30)

Debates may become gradually packaged over time. That is, as portions of an argument or as ways of arguing become standardized, the debate increasingly comes to resemble the exchange of packages whose components are tightly bound together. The contents may be relatively unexamined. For example, there was a great deal of argument in the nineteenth century about the relative merits of induction current versus alternating current in testing electrical responses in the brain (see Ferrier 1876; Dodds 1877–78; Duret 1878). That part of the debate was settled with the adoption of commercial electroencephalograms, which set the standard current for measuring brain electricity. Philosophical questions become settled as well. For example, the argument that "correlation is not causation" is now a familiar one to most scientists (though not always attended to). But in the nineteenth century, it was still fairly fresh—an issue whose points were not universally accepted by the scientific community.

Issues in the Debate

In its simplest form, the idea of localization of function in the brain is based on a constant relation between a region and a function: the "speech area" as located in the third frontal convolution, for example. However, it quickly became apparent to both localizationists and diffusionists that such a simple correspondence did not fit the available data. The basis for much of the debate was the existence of this anomaly; it troubled both diffusionists and localizationists. Ferrier was obviously troubled by the relationship between correlation and causation. He resolved the discrepancy by an appeal to general principles:

It is evident from the discrepancy of views thus enumerated that the facts of disease on which they are based are neither uniform nor altogether simple. I will not here attempt an analysis of the individual cases, adduced in favour of this or that hypothesis, but merely apply certain rules which should guide us in forming a decision on these points. Mere frequency, as the records of cerebral disease amply illustrate, is not sufficient to establish direct causal relationship between the obvious lesion and the symptoms exhibited. (1889: 39)

The antilocalizationist Goltz made a similar comment, pointing out that the same functional result could derive from several antecedents:

The fact that the result of the stimulation is so extremely different according to the location of the stimulated point, suggested that the different sections of the cerebrum could be equally different in their functional meaning. But Fritsch and Hitzig also realized that the stimulation method alone would be insufficient to successfully pursue this idea any further. If we see a group of muscles, for example the muscles of the foot, twitch as a result of a stimulation, the nervous system stimulated can be of very different importance. Whether we stimulate the motor nerves, the spinal cord, the brain, or certain sense nerves, in all cases twitches of the foot muscles can be causes. Therefore, I cannot deduce with certainty from the twitching foot muscle caused by the stimulation of a section of the nervous system, what the functional importance of the stimulated organ is. (MacCormac 1881: 219; see also Goltz 1950 [1888]

Panizza made an even more radical statement about the possibilities of inferring function from injury and about the limits of correlation:

What we deduce from the facts is contrary to the theory of localization. Given these considerations, it is clear that the fact of partial sensory and motor paralysis following an injury to the nerve centers can never be brought up as proof that either sensitivity or the instigating principle of movement is located in the injured spot. In order to be used as proof, it would be necessary for no other area to be injured and give rise to the same effects, and for the same effects always to follow the injury of the same area with absolute constancy. (1887:149)

But such constancy was not to be found in the data, he said. Instead, multiple actions could produce the same result:

Not only can the irritation of *any* point on the nervous system give rise to the same morbid phenomena identical to those obtained by irritating areas that are far apart and totally different, but the most varied phenomena can be obtained by irritating the same point: "Very numerous experiences," writes Brown-Séquard, "which confirm the teachings of human pathology have proved to me that producing the same injury in the same area of animals of the same species can give rise, as in men, to an immense variety of effects." (Ibid.)

The reason that "mere frequency is not enough" was both that many of the data were contradictory or unclear and that multiple results could derive from the same experiment (as well as vice versa). In their struggle to explain contradictions (often brought up as part of an attack by diffusionists), localizationists attempted to develop plastic principles that could withstand the exceptional data.

The anomalies about inconstant relations that concerned diffusionists were of two kinds: symptoms with no lesion (as demonstrated by postmortem examination), and lesions/tumors with no symptoms. Brown-Séquard had this to say about inconstancy as disproving localization theory:

A propagation of organic alterations from the seat of an original lesion in the brain can, of course, give rise to symptoms. But we cannot explain the appearance of symptoms in that way in most cases of hemorrhage, of wound, or of softening of the brain, as it requires more time for the propagation of a morbid state to distant parts of the brain than there is between the moment the lesion takes place and of that apparition of symptoms. Even in cases of tumors enlarging slowly, we cannot look upon such a propagation as the essential cause of appearance of symptoms, as there are many cases of tumors in which there is no propagation of a morbid state. (1873b:253)

Brown-Séquard proposed alternate explanations for the appearance of symptoms in the absence of lesions: change in "quantity or quality of blood"; irritation at a distance; or changes in fluid pressure in the spinal cord or elsewhere. He went on to say:

There is no relation whatever between the extent of a lesion in the brain and the symptoms that may be caused by it. If symptoms were due, as is admitted, to the loss of function of the part altered or destroyed in the brain, or to *immediate* effects of the irritation of such a part, there would be a constant relation between them and the diseases, so that the intensity and extent of the symptoms would be in proportion with the intensity and extent of the alteration. (1873b: 257; emphasis in original)

A second, related class of points raised here by Brown-Séquard was that an "immense variety of symptoms in different individuals may be caused by a lesion in one and the same part of the brain" and/or that "the same symptom may originate from the most various lesions" (1873b: 259).

The issue of multiple lesions/similar symptoms or similar symptoms/multiple lesions was a vexing one for localizationists, as were all forms of the "inconstant relation" argument. As the debate progressed and as anomalies of this nature accrued, localizationists relied more and more heavily on the concept of redundancy of functions. This thesis posited that functions are "localized" in multiple areas; there are multiple "centers of control." Horsley, for example, postulated that there are many centers of control, thus spreading localized functions over a broader area, while he still conceived of them as localized: "The little centres, therefore, which preside over this function are dotted all down the spinal cord in each segmental division of it" (1891: 187). (He had put forth this idea some years earlier under the title "On Substitution as a Means of Restoring Nerve Function Considered with Reference to Cerebral Localisation" [1884].)

Here localizationists and diffusionists approached the same anomaly in very different ways, reflecting their different stylistic commitments. The idea of redundancy allowed localizationists to meet and assimilate many diffusionist criticisms yet remain within an atomistic framework. Redundancy was still a localizationist concept: instead of one center per function, there were many, redundant, centers. By contrast, holistic or distributed functions would mean that different sections of the brain would have part of a function. The function would be distributed over a broad area, with no area being entirely responsible for one function. Yet both localizationists and diffusionists agreed on the existence and importance of the anomaly.

Brown-Séquard was also fascinated with what he saw as a fatal flaw in the localizationist model of the relations of structure and function. One can favor a right hand or a stronger muscle, he suggested, but this does not mean that the function performed by the hand or muscle is what we would today call "hardwired." For him, then, localization was indeterminate as well as inconstant (1873a: 120). So far as I know, this criticism was never addressed by the localizationists in the nineteenth century. Learning and tendencies to perform in a certain way were seen as habits or "impressions" on the nervous system from "accumulated experiences" in the manner of association psychology (Ferrier 1876). This is perhaps a result of triangulation, as discussed in Chapter 4. The atemporal, nondevelopmental approach was developed by localizationists as a result of combining different time horizons and different units of analysis.

Localizationists and diffusionists, then, did not disagree about the existence of symptoms, nor did they even have discrepant views about an ideal one-to-one correlation between function and region, which a strict localization theory would posit. Instead, it was the significance attributed to discrepancies and symptoms by the two camps that differed. Nor were there large differences in the methods used by diffusionists and localizationists to examine these questions. Ferrier, Yeo, Horsley, Brown-Séquard, and Goltz, for example, all used vivisection. They deleted regions of the brain or nervous system, or they produced lesions, to observe the consequences on an organism's behavior. Moreover, all of the debaters relied on patient case histories as sources of data.

The use of debating tactics was similarly comparable across camps. The primary difference in outcome of the debate is thus found not in the superior arguing style of localizationists but in the fact that they were able to link their tactics with a successful organizational enterprise and to embed their theories in multiple, semi-overlapping enterprises.

Although the basis for success here was not purely rhetorical, the rhetoric of the debate is an excellent road map for understanding the *evolution* of the concepts of localization theory and the ways in which localizationists incorporated diffusionist criticisms. In this sense, the debate adds another aspect to the understanding of robustness examined in previous chapters.

Tactics Used in the Debate

Tactics may be used to shift the level of a discussion down to a simpler, perhaps technological point or up to higher moral or philosophical grounds. Upshifting raises the evaluation level of the problem: "It's not as simple as that; it's a question of basic approach." Downshifting lowers the evaluation: "It's not all that complex or important, it's simply a matter of redoing the figures or resetting the electrodes."

Debating tactics can be used at any stage of research: making an argument, challenging it, responding. As positions acquire inertia and momentum and become cumulatively reified, the stage at which debaters apply tactics is significant. A wide range of tactics were employed in the localization debate: to demonstrate facts, analyze inconsistencies, examine or criticize procedures, and identify which skills should be brought to bear to solve the problems. Diplomatic tactics were used to smooth over conflict between negotiators and, at least temporarily, to achieve peace. Other tactics were not so conciliatory, such as the use and abuse of claims that one's argument was superior by virtue of one's status, and all the familiar forms of *ad hominem* argument.

Arguments for the status quo, or appeals to the established nature of a position, were common in the debate. Debaters also attempted to change the configuration of what was significant or insignificant in an argument by switching parts of arguments from foreground to background, or vice versa. They also used their alliances (both interorganizational and intraorganizational) to provide credibility to support or attack an argument. In the next section, I analyze different groups of tactics and their consequences.

Diplomacy

Diplomacy was used to defuse a challenge or as an attempt to establish a competing perspective without antagonizing the "powers that be." Diplomatic tactics included assimilating parts of challenges; creating truisms; and asking audiences to "bear with us."

Assimilating Parts of Challenges

Localizationists often appeared to accept a criticism as true, but then they would not integrate that "truth" into practice. Giving a pro forma acknowledgment to a challenge (often the accusation that data contain artifacts) in the beginning of an article may in practical fact make it easier to ignore the criticism. These bows in the direction of an anomaly are common in scientific research. The scientific community develops a general idea that certain phenomena should, in principle, be accounted for and certain practices avoided. But no mechanism exists for actually changing work practices. For instance, many experimental psychologists today acknowledge that "experimenter expectations" influence research results, or that the laboratory setting creates certain compliance demands for subjects (Orne 1962; Rosenthal 1963, 1966; Star and Gerson 1987). Yet institutionalized methods for accommodating these are rare. We find a similar situation in the claim for *ceteris paribus* in modern clinical trials (Lilienfeld 1982).

Certain anomalies achieved this status in the localizationist-diffusionist dispute. Although localizationists transformed, ignored, or assimilated many diffusionist criticisms, others were taken seriously enough to be openly acknowledged in localizationist writings—but only as disclaimers or truisms. These statements commonly took the form of acknowledging an underlying truth to diffusionism but of judging it to be unimplementable. Thus it was generally acknowledged that the brain was an interrelated whole. Moreover, localizationists talked openly of uncertainty and the imprecision of measurement techniques, though they often blamed error on a different line of work.

The disclaimer about the interrelatedness of the brain took the

form, "Of course we understand that everything's related, but . . . ."
The ellipses implied that such an interrelationship was impossible to
translate into practical action, that it was ineffable, and that it had no
practical implications. Horsley expressed the concept in this way:

Conceivably every part of the body is represented in every nerve-centre, just
as it of necessity is in the single primordial ovum; and that when the nervous
system, considered functionally, is regarded, in the view of Flourens, as working as a whole, the determination of action by any given part is never more
than relative. . . . When we are labouring with the difficulties of endeavoring
to establish a differential diagnosis, we are likely to forget that the whole machine is in active operation while our attention may be drawn to one point
only. (Paget 1919: 180–81)

Horsley wisely noted that the exigencies of clinical diagnosis may
form the de facto elision between theory and practice. Ferrier, by contrast, lodged a disclaimer about the gap in the evolutionary scale:

As we ascend the animal scale, the centres of which the cerebro-spinal system
is composed become more and more intimately bound up and associated with
each other in action, so that to separate the one from the other involves such
functional perturbation of the whole, that only in rare instances is it possible
to obtain indication of independent activity in the part of those which are
not directly injured. (1876: 38)

Later in the same volume, he stated:

The difficulties of localisation necessarily increase when the regions of the
brain under exploration are incapable of being clearly freed from surrounding
sensitive structures; and where such is the case the phenomena must be regarded as of doubtful significance unless their nature can be resolved by other
and complementary methods of investigation. (p. 148)

This last statement of Ferrier's indicated localizationism's view of diffusionist models as true but irrelevant. Diffusionists, in his view, did
not share the same exigencies of clinical practice as did localizationists.

Creating Truisms

Another tactic was to assert that the *basic* premises of the opposing
position were quite true, but only up to a point. Implementing such

premises would be absurd. This tactic sidestepped direct confrontation at the level of basic assumptions; instead, it substituted criteria
of practicality.

A good example of this can be found in Ferrier's *The Localisation
of Cerebral Disease* (1878b). On page 2 he stated that one clear case of
destruction of an area with no resulting functional disorder "would
be sufficient to overturn our conclusion" (about localization), and
two paragraphs later he said:

The doctrine of cerebral localisation does not assume, as Brown-Séquard
would seem to imply, that the symptoms observed in connection with a cerebral lesion are necessarily the result of derangement of function in the part
immediately affected. Everyone admits direct and indirect results in cerebral
disease. We have no right even to assume any causal relation at all, direct or
indirect, between the phenomena, unless the lesion in question is constantly,
or more frequently than chance would account for, associated with the same
symptoms.

Yet, some pages later, he attacked Brown-Séquard for positing an intermediate link between lesions and dysfunctions, and for challenging
the direct link in fact posited by localizationists between lesions and
dysfunctions (pp. 41–42).

The phrase "everyone admits direct and indirect results in cerebral
disease" is a good example of the use of truism as a debating tactic.
Although everyone may have *admitted* that such a phenomenon could
in principle exist, only the diffusionists took serious practical account
of it at the time that Ferrier's article was written. Yet the statement in
some sense is meant to cover the bases against criticism. Goltz made
a similar disclaimer in his discussion:

When these and other considerations forced the conclusion upon me that the
hypotheses of Hitzig, Ferrier and their successors could not possibly be correct, then this did not exclude, of course, the possibility that some totally
different kind of spatial distribution of the functions of the cerebrum does
actually exist. In fact, I have been said (blamed) to deny any localization of
the functions of the cerebrum, but that is wrong. I absolutely believe it possible that the individual cortexes of such a powerful organ as the cerebrum
have varying functions. But whether and how far this possibility proves true,
that will still have to be investigated, dispassionately investigated. (Mac-
Cormac 1881: 223)

Both the localizationists and diffusionists, then, used truisms or partial acceptance of the other's opinions (though Goltz's acceptance was more highly qualified than Ferrier's). Such trusims have the advantage of making the debater appear reasonable, compassionate to the other side's position. It is politically more strategic to offer an alternative explanation than to argue basic premises from scratch. Here we see both sides trying to portray themselves as arguing for alternatives rather than for whole new frameworks.

Another use of truisms appears in the form: "Accept *x*, and *y* follows absolutely," where *x* is taken to be self-evident. Brown-Séquard, for example, made the following claims:

We must admit that either half of the brain can will and regulate the movements of the limbs on the two sides, and that when disease exists in any part of the brain . . . the lesion can produce paralysis either in the corresponding side, and also that if paralysis is produced (I say if—because paralysis is not constant), it is not by the destruction of either the organ of the will or that of conduction between it and the muscles, but by an inhibitory or arresting (or suspensory) influence exerted on distant parts by the irritation of the diseased fibres or cells. If we accept these views . . . then everything becomes clear and easy to explain. (1873c: 142)

"Bear with Us"

Some diplomatic debaters plead with an audience to wait for the future payoff of a set of experiments or the application of a perspective and to accept the basic premises in the meantime. That is, though results cannot be demonstrated now, there is a promise that they soon will be. In one sense, this tactic is an attempt to inveigle an audience into a side bet with the experimenters. Such tactics involve using the unknown to argue for a position. Horsley, for example, made the following statement:

As yet this hypothesis has to be tested by experiments directly bearing on the point, such, for instance, as first extirpating a motor centre completely . . . and then some weeks or months later exploring the portion of brain in the immediate neighborhood with very weak induced currents. . . . But even in the absence of direct experimentation, it is obvious that there are certain centres in the cortex destruction of which, or the fibres leading from them, is followed by permanent paralysis. (1884: 7)

Both sides used the "bear with us" tactic. Some of the most acrimonious aspects of the debate occurred when this tactic was challenged. Atkins (1878) provided an example of ridicule combined with "bear with us," including "don't bear with them." First, he stated that if Brown-Séquard's findings were accepted, then one of the basic findings about the nervous system, the principle of contralateralization, would have to be abandoned. This is familiar to us as the idea that the right half of the brain controls the left half of the body, and vice versa:

These views of M. Brown-Séquard are, comparatively speaking, but recently promulgated; and should they have any foundation, not only the more modern doctrines of localisation, but also the older and hitherto firmly believed in theory of the crossed action of the cerebral hemispheres must be at once and for ever abandoned. (p. 415)

He went on, with elaborate courtesy, to add:

With all respect, however, for their great originator, I hold that we cannot accept these views with the degree of proof at present forthcoming. . . . However, they are now at the bar of science, and time and further research will show sooner or later whether they shall stand or fall. . . . These hypotheses [of localizationists], though they may satisfy the mind for a time, are after all mere speculations which do not throw any real light on the subject. We must be content at present with recording such cases; and, although we may be led to speculate thereon, we can only hope that extended research into now hidden domains may in time afford the real explanation which is at present concealed from our view. (pp. 415–17)

Diplomatic tactics sidestep direct confrontation. One important outcome of diplomacy is that apparent agreement—détente—may be reached on a temporary basis. This cooperation without consensus holds for a period of time, during which different sides compete for resources, establish programs, and continue to argue on other grounds. It can thus be a holding strategy that forestalls confrontation while validity is established through other channels.

Compiling Credibility

Aspects of what we think of as routine scientific practice can also become debating strategies. The persistent compilation of a track record filled with examples or cases is an important tactic in a long debate. Some aspects of this process have received little attention, and I focus on them here.

A tactic called "filtering for exemplars" means emphasizing the examples that most clearly fit one's own side of the theory. I discussed this tactic briefly in Chapter 3, where it was part of constructing clinical, case-based arguments and managing uncertainties encountered in clinical work. Such exemplars construct a smooth match between theory and cases, ignoring contradictory or vague cases that do not fit either taxonomically or diagnostically.

Localizationists presented such exemplars as "celebrated cases." There were several especially dramatic cases in the medical literature, including the first brain tumor operation (Bennett and Godlee 1884) and the first operation for a tumor of the spinal cord by Gowers and Horsley in 1879 (Paget 1919). These were used to underscore the validity of localization, whereas unsuccessful or vague brain or spinal cord tumor cases often went unreported (see National Hospital Records 1870–1901).

Stubbornness can also be an effective strategy for establishing credibility. Many localizationists simply kept on going in an unswerving fashion despite criticism and contradictory evidence. They continued to publish results, repeating analyses with small incremental changes or just slightly varying the application of a formula. Many of the localizationists outlived their opponents, and they essentially buttressed their arguments by compiling case after case over the years.

Brown-Séquard's challenges, for example, spanned two decades, from the early 1870's until his death in 1894. Ferrier, and others to follow, continued to publish books and articles that classified regions of the brain in various animals and humans both during Brown-Séquard's life and after his death (see, for example, Ferrier 1878b, 1910). Despite use of diplomatic tactics and partial assimilation of Brown-Séquard's criticisms, perhaps the most effective tactic of all was the patient repetition of the localizationist argument.

In the clinical sphere, this persistence took shape as the painstaking accrual of cases. Cases of brain damage, stroke, or tumors were presented in medical journals as evidence. These cases, representing a substantial percentage of the journals, were often presented with no explicit theoretical accompaniment or simply with a statement of the form, "*x* symptom indicates functional disturbance in *z* area" (see, for example, Atkins 1878; MacKenzie 1878). The cases were sometimes accompanied by postmortem information showing softening or malformation of the brain in the correctly localized area.

The cases were extremely detailed, often with hour-by-hour descriptions of patient behavior, symptoms, and medication prescribed as well as minute detail about tumors, discharges, and other clinical phenomena. The cumulation of cases here acted as a data base for theoretical arguments as well as a body of evidence composed of numerous examples.

Manipulating Hierarchies of Credibility

A hierarchy of credibility refers to the differential weight given to the word of people or organizations with different status. That is, a person or institution at the top of a hierarchy is intrinsically more "believable" than someone at the bottom (Becker 1967). All else being equal, the word of a Nobel prize winner is likely to be taken as more plausible than that of a vagrant, even if the content of the statements is the same.

Scientific arguments that manipulate hierarchies of credibility are not sanctioned by scientific method. Yet they are common. The localization debate was not won because localizationists were more sarcastic or *ad hominem* than diffusionists. Instead, localizationists could more effectively manipulate hierarchies of credibility as they gained professional power in medicine and physiology.

"More Scientific Than Thou"

Among the types of claims that manipulate hierarchies of credibility are claims on the part of one side or another to scientificity. These are claims that one procedure or approach is more scientifically viable, or technically astute, than another. Such claims are often opposed to designations like "metaphysical," "poetic," "impressionistic," or "soft science." Claims to scientificity are often used in conjunction with new technologies whose drawbacks may not be well understood. Simply to use new technology is thought to be more "scientific" than the employment of older, seemingly less sophisticated methods.

Localizationists often made such claims tacitly as they sought to make medical science more scientific through physiological research. Localizationists claimed to be more scientific than diffusionists by making alliances with doctors using electrical therapies (Schiller 1982) and with evolutionary biologists (Sharpey-Schafer 1927) as well as by using new technologies in histology and microscopy.

Ad hominem arguments should be included in the discussion of hierarchies of credibility, although they pervade many other aspects of the tactics discussed in this chapter. *Ad hominem* tactics criticize an argument on the basis of personal characteristics of the author; they discredit the opponent, attempting to establish that opponent's place as lower in the hierarchy of credibility. These arguments can be subtle or explicit. The localizationist W. J. Dodds, for example, said that "Goltz's results have not been confirmed" whereas Ferrier's results are "far more accurately described than Brown-Séquard's" (1877–78: 361). Ferrier went further; he questioned Brown-Séquard's data and even his ability to interpret them: "Every physiologist who has seen paralysis produced by cerebral lesion, has seen it on the opposite side, with the single exception, I believe, of Brown-Séquard" (1878b: 10). *Ad hominem* discrediting also appeared in a choice of words that added doubt to the actions of opponents. Ferrier used the following phrases in his criticism of Brown-Séquard: "Certain *remarkable* views *advanced* by Dr. Brown-Séquard . . ."; He *professes* to have collected . . ."; ". . . the paralysis from brain disease, he *attributes*, not as is *usually* held . . ." (1876: 233; emphasis added).

Ferrier's summary comment about Brown-Séquard's argument, which Ferrier was trying to discredit, was "I have little to add in the way of comment on these views, beyond the various facts and arguments adduced in the above chapter" (1876: 233).[3] He thus combined *ad hominem* argument with a truism or an appeal to "what should have been obvious" by then to a presumed audience.

Panizza used *ad hominem* argument to impugn localizationists and to argue that their observations were biased by their hypotheses: "In other words, the physiologist sees in these facts which always stay the same, what is convenient to him or what he chooses to see" (1887: 153).

But when referring to diffusionists, Panizza explained anomalous data as due to technical error or carelessness:

Goltz himself admits that it [the dog] made defensive movements analogous to those of the frog to whose skin acetic acid was applied. We have repeated numerous times this experiment and have reached totally opposite results, which, in order not to negate Goltz's statements, forces us to think that he made the experiment only one time, and that in this time, as an exception, the shock of decapitation had immobilized the animal, or had greatly handicapped its sensori-motor reactions. (1887: 153)

Another example of *ad hominem* argument is given by Julius Althaus, who explained disagreements with localizationists psychologically:

As at the present day any opposition to the main features of Broca's theory proceeds only from those who are wilfully blind or disingenuous, the least that the adherents of that doctrine have a right to ask for from their opponents is a thoroughly complete description of the cases brought forward, with the view of disproving the same. (1880: 63)

Here again there is a combination of tactics: *ad hominem* ("must be wilfully blind or disingenuous"); truism ("any opposition to the main features"); and asking for a complete and detailed scientific accounting from opponents.

Arguments from Authority

Another use of the hierarchy of credibility is to argue from authority: to use a political position to one's own advantage. These are manipulations of the hierarchy of credibility to legitimate an argument apart from its technical merits. Such claims can be made through a subtle use of language to describe someone's actions: "Hughlings Jackson *pointed out that* certain convulsions *were due to* disease causing localized irritation on opposite sides. . . . *From such facts he came to the conclusion* that . . ."; "Fritsch and Hitzig *established* that direct current on hemispheres caused movements" (Ferrier 1876: 126–27, 128; emphasis added).

"Pointed out that" casually conveys that Jackson simply noticed a phenomenon and brought it to public attention. Once he noticed these facts, he inevitably came to further conclusions about localization. Similarly, the term "established" in conjunction with the observations of Fritsch and Hitzig tries to put their theory beyond a doubt.

Ignoring, Censorship, and Sarcasm

Other tactics pass over arguments or criticisms, or ignore the opponents themselves (such as neglecting to invite them to professional meetings or to cite their work). Similarly, censorship invokes moral criteria in order to screen opponents' results from publication or discussion. There is an implicit manipulation of the hierarchy of credibility here, because the censors identify themselves with the higher moral status, and therefore with truth.[4]

Sarcasm takes a piece of work, argument, or challenge and implies that it is missing contextual information, that it is "out of place." Sarcastic tactics are often coupled with *ad hominem* arguments—not only is the work "out of place," but the author is "out of it" and misbegotten as well. Although in general the localization debate was imbued with an elaborate courtesy ("with all due respect to my extremely eminent colleague"), debaters sometimes became sarcastic. Brown-Séquard referred to his opponents as "these clever physiologists" 1890a), and Ferrier portrayed his opponents as making an obvious, rather foolish mistake: "What, it is triumphantly asked, could more conclusively dispose of the view that the cortex is concerned in the results, seeing it may be removed without prejudice to them? Apparently, those who argue in this manner forget that there is a plurality of causes and conditions" (1878b: 18).

"Triumphantly" and "apparently" try to undermine diffusionist credibility, and Ferrier's appeal to the obvious further ridiculed his opponents' ideas. Ferrier attempted to convey that *his* ideas were simply what everyone admits; Brown-Séquard's, by contrast, were beyond the pale.

Brown-Séquard used similar tactics. For example: "*It is evident that* hemiplegia as considerable as exists in the case, could not have been caused by the *insignificant* expression that existed in the *pretended* motor centers, and *one must admit* that trephining was followed by recovery because it effected a cessation of the irritation" (1890b: 768; my translation, emphasis added). He attempted to establish certainty and to diminish the importance of the influence of the areas claimed for localization by using words like "insignificant" and "pretended." "One must admit" is also a truism—an attempt to rely on common knowledge, an appeal to the evident, and a tacit attempt to establish the evident.

Much of the stylistic conflict between localizationists and diffusionists was tacit. For localizationists, there was something fundamentally "correct" in an aesthetic that would allocate each function to a discrete place in the brain. One result of different stylistic commitments was an exaggerated perception of the tenets of opponents' theories, resulting in sarcastic or vastly simplified portrayals of those positions.

Diffusionists tended to caricature localizationism as "neophrenology" and localizationists as engaged in an absurd search for separate "organs" in the brain. Similarly, localizationists caricatured diffusionism. First, they portrayed diffusionism as the total collapse of any categorical distinctions (as Goltz complains above, p. 128). Phenomena that, for diffusionists, were distributed through the body or were interactive, were characterized by localizationists as one big chaotic mess. Second, localizationists characterized diffusionism as tautologous: if everything is connected, they argued, then how can anything be said to cause anything else?

Organizational Tactics

Organizational tactics rely on strengthening organizational relationships (or, conversely, on weakening other relations) to advance an argument. Included are *alliances against a common enemy*—that is, the union of two groups of scientists such that attacking the argument of one group becomes an attack on the other. This alliance may disregard the intellectual connections between the two arguments. Similarly, the grounds for enmity become generalized to all work done by "the other side."

What comes to be seen as *logically* necessary connections are thus formed through organizational intersections or professional alliances. As we saw in Chapters 2 and 3, these connections influence the acceptance of arguments and so become debating tactics in their own right.

Other kinds of organizational tactics can be found in the selective enforcement of standards of good scientific practice. Those in power (such as referees, hiring committees, journal editors, and reviewers) use this tactic to help legitimate or impugn arguments.

Controlling the Focus of the Debate

Some tactics push favorable evidence up front and deemphasize unfavorable evidence. The foreground/background relationship of data, or the significance of certain findings, may also be manipulated.[5] The tactics discussed below include the management of anomalies and manipulating public images of theories.

The management of anomalies by alternating between domains of evidence—as described in Chapter 4—can also be used in debate. Overlapping domains of evidence are tapped to circumvent the problems posed by the complex, interactive nature of the brain. In the context of the debate between localizationists and antilocalizationists, this may appear as "passing the buck" or *pro forma* nods in the direction of artifacts. Yet on a practical basis the context of work forming these debates was such that there was neither time nor resources to survey all problem-solving options. Faced with multiple, conflicting problems and demands, researchers made tradeoffs that would resolve as many problems as possible, as elegantly as possible.

Advertising

Scientists often practice what can be called advertising. Advertising in this sense puts one's arguments or results before an audience in the best possible light. The purpose is to obtain the audience's support (financial or otherwise) in a way that disparages opposition and claims to be the best deal. Consider, for example, this editorial from the *British Medical Journal*:

The earnest study of brain function (localization) can hardly fail also to lead to the elucidation of some of the most difficult and interesting physical, educational and social questions. From whatever side it may be viewed—with regard to the treatment of insanity, the diagnosis and treatment of nervous diseases, the solution of the questions of psychology, sociology, and metaphysics—an exact knowledge of the functions of the brain is indispensable. (1881: 823)

This advertisement for the localizationist position claims that it will solve a multitude of problems and be exact, or "clearly" true.

Substituting Precision for Validity

Localizationists sometimes responded to local uncertainties by focusing on the technical precision of their results rather than on their inherent validity. That is, given a bewildering array of problems and pressures, and given a slippery set of criteria for measurement and validation, they often responded by carving out a manageable problem and focusing on precise measurement and description. This substitution also sometimes appeared as a response to technical criticisms of localizationists.

Throughout the debate, there were arguments about the technical adequacy of localizationist and diffusionist experiments and techniques. At times these arguments were used to attempt to discredit one stance or the other; at other times they simply appear to have been arguments within a position about the correct way to go about business.

One common technical artifact raised by both diffusionists and localizationists concerned the use of electrical current (Ferrier 1878a, 1878c). Burdon-Sanderson, for example, attacked the conclusions of Fritsch and Hitzig, "demonstrating to his satisfaction that the results were due to spread of current to the striatum then considered a motor ganglion" (Walker 1957; Burdon-Sanderson 1873–74). Hitzig similarly criticized Ferrier's results as being "vitiated by diffusion currents" (Dodds 1877–78), as did Henry Duret, a French physiologist (Duret 1878).

This criticism was later tested by two Italian localizationist physiologists, Luciani and Tamburini, who, according to a report in *Brain*, determined that "It is absolutely impossible that movements produced by electrisation of the cerebral cortex can be due to diffusion of the current to the dura mater" (Rabagliati 1879: 535). They put glass between the cortex and the dura mater, passed electrical current through both, and then measured the difference. But other criticisms, such as that raised by Foster (1877) and Burdon-Sanderson (Dodds 1877–78), stated that perhaps the currents were electrifying structures deeper in the brain, not in the dura mater.

Two dimensions of this technical debate are important. First, the object of inquiry—the brain and its reactions—is itself labile, reactive to electrical current in some unknown degree, and not uniform in reactions between subjects. Thus the debate about how far the current extends, what kind of current the brain reacts to, and what a response is (as opposed to what an artifact is) meant managing these various uncertainties.

Second, whereas diffusionists struggled to make the artifact significant and thus to impeach localizationism (on grounds of *validity*), localizationist researchers successfully controlled the focus of the argument on issues of precision and reliability. The technical arguments raised by diffusionists were converted to internal procedural arguments.

Arguments within a position can serve to strengthen that position when basic assumptions remain unquestioned, as analyzed in Chapter 3. The focus on a number of second-order problems and on technical details can force a de facto resolution of ultimate stylistic or political commitments. Such is the case with several of the technical artifacts raised in the localization dispute, especially those, like electricity, whose uses were an unquestioned part of medical practice. The management and manipulation of focus was important in accomplishing this substitution.

Referencing the Unknown

Another way of managing the focus of the arguments was to invoke the unknown, or some putative future results, in order to support one's side. This means that unsolvable problems could be referred to nonempirical or extremely remote domains so that the immediate argument could continue. For example, Ferrier, in discussing the problem of indeterminacy of lesion-function relationships, attacked Brown-Séquard for using as-yet-unknown results to establish his point of view:

Owing, however, to the fact, as Hughlings Jackson has remarked, that "the damage by disease is often coarse, ill-defined, and widespread," the determination of the functions of the brain by the clinicopathological method had made comparatively little progress, there being apparently no constant uniformity between the seat of the disease and the symptoms manifested. The difficulty of discriminating between the direct and indirect effects of cerebral lesions had furnished Brown-Séquard with arguments in favour of his peculiar views, that all the symptoms of cerebral disease are due to some dynamic influence exercised by the lesion on parts situated at a distance (and always apparently out of reach), which are credited with the functions lost or otherwise disturbed. (1890: 15–16)

"Always apparently out of reach" was Ferrier's sarcastic objection to Brown-Séquard's use of the as-yet-unknown results of research. Brown-Séquard posited an influence at a distance whose nature or location was unknown; localizationists referred to unseen but probable tumors. Both used these unknown or unverifiable entities to prove a point. (Hornstein and Star, forthcoming, discuss the use of such "invisible referents" in marketing theories about human nature.) This was not simply speculation, in the sense of propositions that might have been true; instead, it extended a conceptual framework to unprovable realms. Brown-Séquard gave an example of this in localizationist work:

Lesions of a very small part of the brain often produce very marked symptoms. . . . It is evident that the old theory of production of symptoms of brain disease (localization) is absolutely unable to explain such facts. The only way to get out of the difficulty is to suppose that the autopsy has not been well made, and that a lesion, not discovered, existed somewhere else than the one found, and that this supposed lesion was the cause of the symptoms. It is, of course, quite possible, if not certain, that real organic lesions have frequently escaped notice;[6] but it would be a purely gratuitous supposition to admit that it always has been so in the very large number of cases in which only a small lesion has been found in the cerebral lobes in the bodies of persons who had had decided symptoms of brain disease. (1873b: 254–55)

Ferrier attacked Goltz for the same type of logic:

The results of ablation of the cerebral hemispheres indicate nothing for or against the doctrine of functional localisation, nor do the experiments of Goltz in the least degree militate against the existence of specific centres; for if, even after complete bilateral extirpation of these centres, the functions which survive do not transcend those capable of being manifested in the entire absence of the cerebral hemispheres, there still remains the question whether the lesions have not caused a loss or paralysis of something of a higher order. That this is so is capable of ample demonstration, of which not the least part has been contributed by the very facts which Goltz himself has ascertained through the numerous and varied devices which he has so ingeniously contrived. It is no explanation of the defects which admittedly result from removal of the cerebral hemispheres to say that they are caused by a loss of intelligence. This is merely restating the facts in a more metaphysical but less intelligible form. We are not, however, dealing with metaphysical terms when we are studying the effects of lesions of the cerebral cortex. We are dealing with material entities connected with sensory and motor tract, and it is our object to determine, if possible, what are the anatomical and physiological factors which are correlated with the functions which we generalise under the head of intelligence. (1890: 13)

Both sides here accused one another of the same sin: using the unknown to resolve anomalies or extend frameworks. Such uses were labeled "metaphysics" by Ferrier and "gratuitous supposition" by Brown-Séquard.

Another form of controlling focus emphasized inconsistencies or uncertainties in the opponent's data or procedures while ignoring one's own. These may have been inconsistencies or uncertainties to which the opponent admitted, but the debating tactic emphasized them as more significant than the positive results obtained.

This was common when the diffusionist/localizationist debate included demonstrations of experimental or clinical findings. In nineteenth-century medicine and physiology, arguments were often supplemented with public demonstrations. Such demonstrations used all of the tactics of a dramatic setting. An example from the clinical work of the Queen Square neurologist Gowers vividly illustrates the ways in which dramatic techniques were used to focus aspects of arguments:

His [Gowers's] teaching clinics soon became thronged with physicians from all over the world standing in the gangways and straining the capacity of the accommodation. Gowers was able to combine teaching with out-patient consultations, and he set the practice which has been followed ever since. He was not aware beforehand of what cases were attending and he saw the patient for the first time in the presence of a critical and admiring audience. He took the history, examined the patient, and afterwards discussed the nature of the case, the differential diagnosis, prognosis and treatment. There was no set talk; no questions or answers. . . . If clinical cases were to be shown, careful arrangements were made beforehand with his house physician. Gowers was well aware of his skill as an instructor, and was even guilty of a certain justifiable vanity in respect of his powers of attracting large audiences. (Critchley 1949: 81–82)

Here, the patient's disease was used to instantiate a taxonomy of disease based on localization theory (see Gowers 1885). With this form of argument—example-giving—there was little time or space for rebuttal or counterargument on an analytic level. The focus in this case was managed so that all diagnoses appeared to be successful ones and to support the taxonomic framework being developed by the Queen Square physicians.

Another kind of demonstration occurred at medical congresses and other professional meetings. The famous confrontation between Ferrier and Goltz at the 1881 International Medical Congress (MacCormac 1881) included an exhibition of each man's experimental animals. Each was literally given the stage for a set period of time, and each made his point by offering material, publicly observable evidence (see pp. 104–5 in this volume for details of the confrontation). The experimental animals were later killed, and a blue-ribbon committee of anatomists and physiologists determined if the dogs were indeed decorticate and if the monkey's injuries were in fact limited to the areas Ferrier claimed as damaged. A report of this investigation was published two years after the conference in the *Journal of Physiology* (Klein, Langley, and Schafer 1883–84). This delay probably reflected the slowness of the dissection process at the time; it took nearly eighteen months to perform a full histological examination of a brain.

A critical aspect of convincing an audience is precisely the length of time it can take to refute a demonstration or instantial argument of this form. In this case, Ferrier had the upper hand in several ways. When the proceedings were published a few months after the conference (MacCormac 1881), Goltz's remarks were not translated from the German, either in the proceedings or, presumably, at the conference itself. Ferrier's animals were demonstrated last, after Goltz had presented his dogs. Thus the "final word" was Ferrier's.

Arguing for the Status Quo

Arguing for the status quo includes claims that changing procedures or disconfirming results would endanger precious resources. This tactic often turns into appeals to tradition. For example, this review from *Brain* characterized Brown-Séquard as denying "all scientific progress": "The hypothesis of Brown-Séquard, who denies the possibility of localising in the cortex or any other part of the brain functions of any kind, besides being a denial of all scientific progress, is contradicted by experimental and clinical results, and the facts brought to sustain his book are not of a kind to destroy the doctrine of localisation" (Rabagliati 1878b: 145).

Another example of this tactic appears in the following bitter criticism of Brown-Séquard made by Ferrier:

> Brown-Séquard, however, holds that, in all cases of paralysis from cortical lesion, there is some intermediate link or *tertium quid* intervening between the antecedent and the consequent: a kind of inhibitory influence exerted by the lesion on some centre or centres which are credited with those functions which are lost. It would, I think, be easy by parity of reasoning—and I say it with all due respect to the distinguished author of this theory—to make a complete *reductio ad absurdum* of the whole of experimental psychology. We should never be entitled to infer direct relationship between organ and function, but be condemned to a perpetual search after some *tertium quid*, which, like an *ignis fatuus*, would for ever elude our grasp. (1878b: 41–42)

Ferrier invoked this argument selectively. Foster had made a similar point in his 1877 text, where he cautioned against simplistic causal interpretations of function loss/area damage. He saw inhibition as an important factor in nervous function and one that could easily be misunderstood (p. 446). Yet Foster agreed with localization, and his *tertium quid* accorded with localization and the logic of deletion.

This tactic, like many, never had a conclusive result. It may have been "wrong" to bring in a *tertium quid* without specifying the nature of the intervening relationship. However, that did not in itself prove that the *tertium quid* did not exert an influence, only that certain rules of argument had not been followed. Ferrier here collapsed the rules of the arguments with ascertaining the validity of the data, a common and fascinating phenomenon in scientific debate.

Modes of Debate and Tacit Debates

The debating tactics used by localizationists and diffusionists were employed in several different modes. Each of these types of argument was tied to the experiences of work and defended from that work. Two major modes were *argument by example* and *argument by comparative taxonomy*.

Instantial arguments fill slots in a framework. For physiologists and physicians trying to map functional regions of the brain, this meant filling in areas on outlines of the brain. The instantial maps were supported by matching movements or disturbances of function with areas in the brain (see, for example, Ferrier 1873–74, 1876).

The "filling in" activity itself in a sense *became* the argument. For instance, Beevor and Horsley (1890, 1894) did a series of experiments on monkeys in which tiny areas of the brain were exposed to electrical current. Movements were then recorded and areas correspondingly labeled. Accompanying the articles' text were plates with representations of the monkey brain, shaded for various localized cortical regions. The explicit part of the work gave information about the movements of these monkeys after being exposed to electrical current. The implicit argument was that the map of their brains had only to be filled in. These example-filled maps were a major product of localizationism (Young 1970: 234).

Beevor and Horsley's first experiment was attacked by Brown-Séquard in an article entitled "Proofs of the Insignificance of a Celebrated Experiment by Victor Horsley and Beevor on the So-Called Motor Centers" (1890a). He offered an alternative explanation for the movements made after the application of current. Just because an electrical current in area *x* made the thumb move, he argued, we cannot conclude that that part of the brain determines thumb movements. Similarly, a person whose face is tickled will always smile; if one used the same logic as Beevor and Horsley, then the "smile center" would be in the facial skin. Brown-Séquard argued: "All reflex movements in the organism would furnish a similar argument against the value of the fact presented by the English physiologists" (p. 199, my translation).

Here, Brown-Séquard used sarcasm to make his point. Later in the article he simply declared the opposition to be wrong, stating:

All the value of the facts of irritation in the so-called motor region of the cerebral cortex, after the experiments of Fritsch and Hitzig, David Ferrier, Horsley and Beevor and of others, are certainly annulled by the experiments demonstrating that the same part of this region on the other side of the brain is capable of producing, under the same conditions, identical movements. (p. 201, my translation)[7]

Brown-Séquard's argument was the same as that used by localizationists to explain why functions are sometimes retained after destruction of an area thought to be responsible. He postulated that two areas (or multiple areas) were capable of producing movement. If this was so, he asked, then why did destruction of both these regions sometimes not cause paralysis? The answer given by Brown-Séquard was that effects were not localized in the motor cortex, but could be caused at a distance in the nervous system, and were either inhibiting or action-producing.

Brown-Séquard was trying to prohibit the localizationists from moving down an instantial hierarchy and simply fitting their examples into a presumed map. He did this by questioning the nature of the hierarchy. He provided an alternative explanatory framework for the phenomenon, and he employed many of the tactics described above (sarcasm, use of truisms, *ad hominem*). The tacit framework was thus challenged and made explicit.

Summary

It is clear from the preceding discussion that both sides in the debate about localization used many kinds of tactics to make their points and that they employed several strategies. Ultimately, however, most of the criticisms raised by the diffusionists were absorbed into the tenets of localization theory. The dynamics of the debate are another part of the fascinating "historical puzzle" to which I referred at the beginning of this book. The process of absorption can be seen as the debate progresses: issues are raised and re-raised, and they move from the status of damaging criticisms to truisms. The very thickness of the debate, the multiple issues that were entangled and often confounded within it, and the many different kinds of tactics used by both sides became sources of stability in the debating arena. "Loyal oppositions" emerged, and both sides acknowledged that parts of the other's point of view were valid. Yet the localizationist side became increasingly dense over the period examined here: each point was linked to several organizational contingencies and work considerations. The diffusionist side, on the other hand, became thinner. Its research programs were never fully realized with the same degree of organization. Although Goltz's work was instrumental in many later developments in neurophysiology, including the work of Sherrington, his fundamental argument with localizationism became incorporated into the localizationist canon.

In the following chapter, I will analyze another aspect of localization theory's growth and entrenchment: the commitment to psychophysical parallelism (mind/brain relationship), its embeddedness in work organization, and how localizationists resolved some of the difficulties posed by this philosophy.

The Mind / Brain Problem: Parallelism and Localization

"Parallelism" is the doctrine that the mind and the body operate as two separate but parallel realms. This idea predated the localizationists; the work of Descartes is commonly cited as exemplary of its first form, and there are earlier instances as well. But the localizationists played an important part in integrating the doctrine of parallelism into modern neurophysiology and medicine. Whereas the mind / body problem is the overall issue, I am concerned here with the more specific mind / *brain* problem—that is, the brain as a physiological entity.

At its heart, research into localization of function implied psychophysical parallelism. That is, for a psychological function to be located in a particular site (as the localizationists conceived of this) meant that two parallel domains had to be joined in some fashion. Without parallelism, there would be no reason to investigate localization. The reverse of this is not true. That is, one could posit that functions are distributed over the brain or body but still inhabit a domain separate from them. It is the fashioning of the conceptual joins between brain and behavior that is the subject of this chapter.

There have been thousands of articles and books on the subject of the relationship between the mind and the brain since the 1870's (see, for example, James 1890; Ryle 1949; Smart 1955; Smith 1959; MacKay 1978; Sperry 1980; Eccles 1982). The philosophical problem is enormously complicated. This is at least in part because of the very different approaches taken by philosophers and neurophysiologists. It is not within the scope or intent of this book to recapitulate those arguments, nor even to try to give a summary of the range of positions.[1] Much of the history of the entire discipline of psychology can be thought of as one long argument about parallelism: where does behavior "come from"? Is it nature or is it nurture? What is the relationship between biology and behavior?

My concern here is with how the work arrangements of neurophysiologists strengthened the commitment to a philosophy of parallelism. This commitment subsequently informed the debate about the relationship between the mind and the brain, and helped it persist.

Localizationists chose parallelism as a philosophical approach from the conditions of their daily work. Their audiences imposed constraints and supplied resources. The success of localizationism and the nature of work practices meant that parallelism would be part of neurophysiological research ever afterwards.

Once committed to parallelism, localizationists faced stringent criticism from philosophers of science and from other researchers (such as James 1881). They were in many senses in an odd position. On the one hand, philosophers of science welcomed the results of localizationist experiments. Many thought that a new kind of solution to old mind / body problems would be found in this work. In this sense, then, localizationists were hailed as philosophical heroes. On the other hand, these men were in fact not full-fledged academic philosophers. They attempted to address the subtle philosophical questions of the mind / body problem in their writings about the brain. In so doing, they often incurred the wrath of philosophers or inadvertently found themselves in the middle of an academic morass.

In facing the criticisms of philosophers, localizationists were forced to construct temporary solutions that allowed them to continue with their work but that did not in fact resolve the philosophical problems. These temporary solutions were plausible bridges between the mind and the brain—but they were makeshift epistemologies.

Parallelism and the Work Situation

In Chapter 4, I discussed the triangulation strategies developed by localizationists to manage the difficulties that arise when two or more ways of measuring the same phenomenon are combined. In creating a common object, researchers often make the assumption that the boundaries of the phenomenon—as established by the several lines

of work—coincide. Surgeons, neurologists, pathologists, and physiologists were all addressing the problem of localization of function
in the nervous system. As their results were used to legitimate one
another's findings, a common boundary for the functions they addressed was (often tacitly) established. The emergence of *coincident
boundaries* here is important in understanding another aspect of the
theory's success and entrenchment. This was the practical resolution
of philosophical conundrums (Wimsatt 1980b).

Localizationists approached the mind/brain relationship from
within the constraints imposed by the materials with which they
worked. Neurologists investigated and treated paralysis, epilepsy, and
various other disorders. Surgeons attempted to locate tumors within
the brain and nervous system; they needed to understand nervous
anatomy in order to avoid serious damage inside the skull. Physiologists observed muscle movements; they made correlations between
the application of electrical current or deletion of an area and such
movements. Pathologists, like surgeons, observed the physical characteristics of the brain, the differential distribution of types of cells,
and the composition of tumor cells.

As localizationists coordinated findings from these different fields
to make their arguments for localization of function, they tacitly
agreed on many things, including *common boundaries* for the phenomena addressed by their several lines of work. These boundaries were
the skull and the skin. Quite simply, these were the physical limits
faced by surgeons and physiologists, who had to cut through them.
They were the informational barriers for neurologists, who had to
guess what was inside and exactly where it was located. The skull and
skin were demarcations of data for pathologists.

Bentley (1975c), in his essay "The Human Skin: Philosophy's Last
Line of Defense," provides a brilliant analysis of the philosophical implications and limits of adopting the skin (and, by extension, the
skull) as a boundary for philosophical analysis. He argues that there
is no logical or analytic a priori for adopting the skin for analyzing
behavior. Nevertheless, we take it for granted that the skin bounds
many kinds of activity. When we view human beings as ending at the
skin, we create an analytic chasm that can never be bridged—not by
interaction, society, history, or knowledge. This is the chasm between
organism and environment in which both are reified. Many questions

about the nature of knowledge get begged because we take the skin for granted as the outer limit: an example of such a lack of knowledge would be the nature of interpersonal communication. Thus the skin as boundary has provided an enduring basis for dualism and physiological reductionism.

Localizationists found themselves facing a similar philosophical chasm. For them, the skull became the edge of the mind; it was the physical boundary for mental functions. (Although it is true that localizationist experimenters also conducted research on the spinal cord, what we think of today as the higher functions they saw as contained within the skull. These included thought, imagination, many kinds of speech, and motor control.) These researchers did say that there was a distinct difference between mental and physical realms, as we shall see below. However, the triangulation of their work results forced them to act as if these realms had a common boundary.

There was support from other sources for the idea that the individual mind was contained in the individual nervous system. Developments in medicine encouraged this view. After the 1860's, the germ theory of disease—coupled with an emphasis on the individual patient—prevailed over group or epidemiological models. Increasingly, investigators focused on diseases as located exclusively inside the individual. I contrast this with the view of disease held by doctors earlier in the century, when they often mixed patients with different diseases within hospital wards so as not to "concentrate" one type of disease in one place. It was thought that so doing might make the disease more powerful. This was not a theory of contagion as we now think of it. Instead, it was an approach to disease that did not take the boundary of the skin for granted; disease was more like the weather than like an event occurring inside separate skins. The growing success of surgery using antisepsis also supported this individualist emphasis. The germ theory of disease strengthened the organism/environment distinction. Germs invaded: when a surgeon opened the skin for surgery, an opening for germs was created. With the skin as a barrier against germs and a barrier to be crossed in the surgical process, the boundary concept was reinforced. Again, the skin became the outer limit for analysis.

As the individual patient became an ever-stronger unit of analysis in medicine, other events influenced the adoption of parallelism by localizationists. E. G. Boring (1950) believed that the localizationists were heavily influenced by association psychology. He stated that this influence was an important reason for the adoption of parallelism. The definition of causality developed by medical thinkers in the mid-nineteenth century, he reasoned, involved simple chains of cause and effect. Coupled with a mechanistic view of the physical world, this causal reasoning gave rise to the localizationist approach. "Bain . . . in the 1870's . . . did not see how a neural event could cause a psychic one without transferring energy to it, nor a psychic event, with no physical energy to give us, cause a neural one. . . . That was the argument which gave victory to parallelism in the late nineteenth century" (pp. 666–67).

Robert M. Young (1970) also believes that the localizationists were directly influenced by the associationists. I find the evidence less striking than he does for a simple, direct influence. Ferrier *was* Bain's student, but this provides an incomplete explanation for linking Ferrier's theories with his actual work. Jackson relied heavily on the work of Spencer in all of his analyses; this is clearly visible throughout his work and letters. By contrast, Ferrier's references to Bain and other associationists are much less clear.

Returning to the contingencies of everyday work, however, there was no doubt that, for the localizationists, physical realms were preferable to mental realms for getting work accomplished. Mental phenomena were messy, imprecise, and not easily discovered or replicated. As Jackson said: "Our concern as medical men is with the body. If there be such a thing as disease of the mind, we can do nothing for it" (1932e: 41).

Wherever possible, localizationists opted for explanatory primacy for the physical realm. The brain caused the mind, and not the other way around. If only they could understand the brain, the mind would follow. Yet they all understood the importance of trying to decipher psychological cues and mental events. Such phenomena could not be dismissed altogether, for they often formed the immediate clues to nervous disease found by the neurologists (see, for instance, Crichton-Browne 1872; Ross 1882a).

Particularly interesting in this regard is the study of aphasia—a complex impairment of speech or language ability. It may range from total muteness to a restricted ability to speak some words, or a distorted speech capacity. Some forms of aphasia are often a symptom of brain disease, though not all inability to speak is aphasia per se; neurologists distinguish it from a simple physical impairment, as with impaired vocal cords, which prevent enunciation. But, to localizationists in the nineteenth century, when the vocal cords were not damaged yet patients were unable to speak, write, or produce or understand language normally, the diagnosis was aphasia. They saw aphasia as a type case of a mental phenomenon caused by physical brain damage (see Seguin 1881).

The fact that there were many types of aphasia (Head 1926; Riese 1977) added to the intrigue and complexity of the problems represented. Some forms of aphasia interfered with the ability to understand words, others with the ability to produce them. Still others were classified as impairments of the ability to talk to oneself, but not of the ability to talk to or understand others.

Localizationists sought to correlate these subtly different impairments with physical damage or brain tumors. As evidence from different realms was accumulated, researchers developed an increasingly strict doctrine of psychophysical parallelism. Again, this was the idea that the brain and the mind operate in tandem but as completely separate and sovereign realms. As the Jackson scholar H. Tristam Engelhardt, Jr., states:

The choice between these options was important, for it would define what factors and indeed what "facts" would be of immediate significance to neurology. For example, a materialism would dismiss the importance of psychological events, while an interactionism would require such events to be acknowledged as causal factors. But a theory of the concomitance of mind and body would allow one to attend to purely physiological explanation without denying the significance of psychological reality. In developing his notion of neurology, Jackson considered that he was making a pragmatic choice between these options. (1972: 23; see also Levin 1960)

Jackson's claims for the separation of the two spheres were quite strong. They were based on the reliability of the physiological parameters: "The trustworthy symptoms in the diagnosis of actual and primary disease of the organs of the mind are physical, and the untrustworthy symptoms for that diagnosis are mental" (1875: 492). Most explicitly, he said that:

The doctrine I hold is: first, that states of consciousness (or, synonymously, states of mind) are utterly different from nervous states; second, that the two things occur together—that for every mental state there is a correlative nervous state; third, that, although the two things occur in parallelism, there is no interference of one with the other. This may be called the doctrine of concomitance. (1932a: 72).

There was another important consequence of the adoption of this doctrine, however, and one that has had a lasting impact on neurology's philosophical dilemmas. This was the fact that localizationists found themselves in an old and tangled arena in the philosophy of science about the relationship between the mind and the brain. Not only were they *in* the arena, but they suddenly became a focal point for it (Calderwood 1879). There is not space here to review the history of the entire arena. However, localizationist neurosurgery and neurology provided entirely new phenomena to examine and a powerful empirical base for explanations of parallelism. Philosophers of science had previously lacked such empirical data. They had not been able to link explanations of the mind/brain relationship with this type of successful clinical program (Ireland 1879).

Thus several factors created a kind of philosophical deadlock about the relationship between the mind and the brain: the adoption of psychophysical parallelism, the close scrutiny from philosophers, the lack of such clear empirical demonstrations for these philosophical ideas, triangulation, and the complex debates about localization. In a sense, this deadlock has persisted to the present day in the neurosciences, and the terms of the debate have also not shifted significantly (see, for example, Wimsatt 1976; Laurence 1977; Schmitt and Worden 1979; Sperry 1980; Eccles 1982).

Localization theory was crucial in helping to define, and subsequently to support, parallelism. The importance of this role can be seen through understanding the nature of the philosophical problems as these researchers conceived of them, including the contradictions they faced and the ways they resolved those contradictions. The following section considers several strategies employed by researchers to resolve philosophical dilemmas.

The Contradictions

Localizationists recognized that material and immaterial realms could not, without serious philosophical difficulties, simply be posited as causing action in one another. They also recognized that in principle "correlation is not causation," although they sometimes used correlation as proof. The major conceptual difficulties thus caused by parallelism were *how* the two realms (mind and brain) were brought together and *by what mechanisms* they were made to operate in tandem. Again, it is not surprising to find that the localizationists' responses to these problems were neither unified nor consistent. They were facing multiple, incommensurate audiences: philosophy, medicine, physiology, antivivisection, and evolutionary biology. In addition, their everyday work posed serious technical difficulties and uncertainties.

In order to resolve the conflicting demands of the several audiences, localizationists adopted several general strategies. The first strategy was to refer philosophical problems to an expert *within their ranks*. This was someone who understood their daily work concerns but who would speak as a philosopher for them. The person elected to do this was John Hughlings Jackson. Because he addressed many of the contradictions posed by parallelism and the mind/brain relationship, Jackson became a kind of symbolic leader for localizationists (Klapp 1964 discusses the concept of symbolic leader more broadly).

The second strategy was to develop theories and concepts that could act as *plausible bridges* between the realms of the mind and the brain. These explanations were not, strictly speaking, philosophically accurate. However, they were good enough as theoretical explanations to allow work to continue respectably.

As a final resort, when problems could not be resolved, localizationists would simply jettison intractable problems into other lines of work. That is, those difficulties that could not easily be addressed by some physical or medical model were relegated to "mind"-related lines of work, such as psychiatry and psychology. In this way, psychophysical parallelism was reinforced on an organizational level. Such a division of labor effectively obscured many of the epistemological problems arising from the mind/brain gap. The contradictions were thus eradicated from immediate concern.

I will consider each of these strategies in turn below.

Jackson as Symbolic Leader

Symbolic leaders are individuals who embody or represent one kind of activity or position in a conflict (Klapp 1964). The participants in a conflict vest such a figure with power to speak for a viewpoint or debating stance. They often invoke her or his image to embody one side or the other of the conflict. (For example, Gloria Steinem is often invoked as a broad reference to feminism, only partly in reference to her actual work.) As Strauss (1961) discusses in his analysis of the images people develop of American cities, social worlds form composite shorthand images that come to have the quality of stereotypes.

There are dozens of testimonial articles, references, and honorifics accorded to Jackson.[2] Many of them attest to Jackson's lasting influence in neurology and neurophysiology: "He is, by general consent, awarded the first place among those who have contributed to neurology as a science, and his stature continues to grow with the passage of time" (Bishop 1960: 4); ". . . the acclaimed Master, the father of British neurology" (Critchley 1960a: 617). Several historian/neurologists refer to Jackson as being "ahead of his time." In part, this refers to the lasting puzzles addressed by localizationists and to Jackson's role as articulator of the puzzles: "Even today we may not have entirely grasped the magnitude of Jackson's ideas, for his intellectual life was a century ahead of his contemporaries" (Critchley 1960b: 9); "John Hughlings Jackson was one of the unique medical scientists of the nineteenth or any other century. Some historians say he was too far advanced for his era. It may be that he has remained such throughout the years, that he conceived a master plan for the study and classification of neurological diseases" (Lassek 1970: 3); "He was ahead not only of his own time, but in some respects of our own" (Brain 1957: 91).

Jackson was also the oldest of the important localizationist theorists. In many ways he formed the key bridge between the older physicians' more diffusionist approaches and the newer localizationism

(Greenblatt 1970). He had been a student of Brown-Séquard's, although they disagreed vehemently about localization. Still, Jackson's language was more familiar to those in the old school: he spoke of forces moving through the body, and of balances, at the same time as he spoke of localization of function. He said, wryly, of himself, "I am neither a universaliser nor a localiser. . . . In consequence I have been attacked as a universaliser and also as a localiser. But I do not remember that the view I really hold as to localisation has ever been referred to" (1932e: 35).

Jackson's medical methods and many other aspects of his theory derived from assumptions and training practices prevalent throughout British medicine. He adhered to many of the older methods of diagnosis and treatment while bringing these methods into the new arena of localization of function.

While at York Medical School, Jackson studied under Thomas Laycock (Lassek 1970).[3] Laycock's *Lectures* on medical methods (1857) provided clear methodological and theoretical precedents for Jackson's work. Throughout that volume, Laycock stressed the *order* of events as of primary importance in medical diagnosis. This concern was later reflected in Jackson's observations of the sequence of events in an epileptic seizure. Laycock, too, emphasized that disease is a deviation from normal, to be measured only in extent of deviation. For Laycock, "A theory is a means to an end only, namely, the progressive discovery of the order of events. . . . [T]he observation of the order of succession of phenomena is the foundation of etiology" (1857: 50, 81).

The generational difference between Jackson and Laycock was a crucial one, however. The differences in their theories were a reflection of the changing medical approaches of the mid-nineteenth century. Laycock was concerned with environmental, extraorganismic factors in disease. He discussed the importance of seasonal, meteorological, cyclic, and temperature changes (1857: 129–32). By Jackson's time, some fifteen to twenty years later, these concerns had almost disappeared except in anecdotal notes in medical records. The organism / environment distinction had become more sharply drawn in medical practice.

Like Brown-Séquard, Jackson is perhaps best known in medicine, then and now, for his work on epilepsy. He described epileptic seizures in great detail and was a pioneer in collecting clinical details about the disease. He created an evolutionary theory about epilepsy, as well as about the whole nervous system (Jackson 1878, 1879). He argued that epilepsy represented, in perfect ordinal correspondence, a process of "dissolution" that was the opposite of evolution. This was a concept directly borrowed from Spencer (see, for example, Jackson 1932a, 1932e), who saw the entire natural and social world in terms of evolution and dissolution. Jackson was a staunch Spencerian throughout his career (Smith 1982).

Many historians of neurology have referred to Jackson as exclusively influenced in theory-making by Spencer. For example, Head (1926: 31) stated that "Jackson derived all his psychological knowledge from Herbert Spencer." Yet as we have seen above, Jackson's work was also an exemplar of contemporary diagnostic forms and a crucial bridge between old and new systems of medicine. Use of Spencer's language proved important in cementing alliances with, and making plausible arguments to, evolutionary biologists. Localizationists and evolutionary biologists and philosophers had become political allies in the antivivisection debates and trials of the 1870's (French 1975). The two groups had formalized many of these professional alliances in the formation of the Physiological Society (Sharpey-Schafer 1927; see also the discussion above, pp. 57–58).

Jackson claimed to be a strict parallelist. His "doctrine of concomitance" stated that the brain (or nervous system) and the mind are two separate realms that act *at the same time* but do not touch. Further, based on the contingencies of work, he believed that physiology was the only proper realm for medical investigation.

But Jackson's claims to strict parallelism, and his attempts to demarcate a strictly physiological sphere of investigation, were not entirely successful (Engelhardt 1975). Jackson was forced to address the philosophical problem of linkage between the realms he distinguished. His writing on the subject was dense, rich with contradictions and subtleties (Mitchell 1960), and it embodied all the complexly interwoven processes described throughout this volume. He wove together clinical and basic evidence, he absorbed anomalous information by incorporating objections and changing their framework into a localizationist-oriented one, and he coupled abstract concerns about the nature of cognition with practical clinical advice based on years of working with epileptics and victims of nervous disorders.

The result is a body of work with many of the attributes of scripture: infinitely interpretable, inspirational, and filled with both hardheaded advice and ambiguity. Jackson's work became the final authority on the mind/brain problem in the same way that any such writing becomes authoritative: it was quoted for a wide variety of purposes, interpreted by many, and, ultimately, became a repository for unanswerable questions. Other researchers could cite his work rather than founder with difficult philosophical questions.

Plausible Bridges

In addition to using Jackson's work as the authority on unanswerable questions, localizationists also formed several kinds of temporary, workable theoretical bridges over the mind/brain chasm.

One such bridge was *concomitance theories*. These were theories based on the correlation of activity between the mind and the body. They lodged the connection in temporal simultaneity. If a tumor was discovered in the brain of a former patient who had aphasia, then the tumor was affecting the speech area. Both speech and the brain were affected at the same time, therefore there must be a connection between the brain (tumor) and the mind (speech). These theories relied heavily on the concept of *substrata*, either anatomical or physiological, that underlie functions or behaviors. The major philosophical difficulty here was with discovering the nature of connections between the presumed substratum and its products. The nature of learning also presented difficulties: how does learning occur, since it involves both a substratum and a behavior.

Building-block theories attempted to find "basic units" whose assembly would constitute either brain or mind. These were theories that conceived of actions as being built up of particulate sets of reflexes. The primary difficulties implied by such reflex theories were problems of storage of nervous impulses and coordination between basic units (Dewey 1981 [1896]).

Representation theories tried to link the realms of mind and brain by positing that one realm "stood for" and indicated or implied the other. These theories were the most abstruse, and much of Jackson's work relied on these sorts of concepts. According to representation theories, the gap between mind and brain was bridged by a kind of calling back and forth, or imaging, between realms. Representation theories included theories of ordinal representation, automaton theories, and some theories about muscle sense. In discussing representations across realms, they also often addressed behavioral problems in terms of consciousness and unconsciousness. A major source of difficulty for these theories was how to account for mechanisms of perception between or across realms: what symbolic "language" could bridge the gap between mind and brain, for example?

A practical concern about the usefulness of concomitance often appeared in the early volumes of the localizationist journal *Brain*, which was founded in 1878. Writers stated therein that, even though the connection between the realms of brain and mind was impossible to understand philosophically, concomitance was the only practical solution to the difficulties. In short, it was a theory that would allow them to get on with their work.[4] This example from James Cappie was typical:

In studying the causation of mental phenomena we need not be deterred by the fact that our knowledge, at the best, is likely to be always remote. It may not be the less positive so far as it may pretend to go. We must ever be content to accept the fact of consciousness as ultimate. The physiologist will never be able to perceive why the brain's activity should be associated with its manifestations. Yet, if a correlation be assumed, he may be able to determine why one form of consciousness rather than another is present; why it is present with a felt amount of intensity; or why in certain circumstances it is obscured or suspended. The nexus between molecular activity of brain and activity of thought and volition may forever remain "unthinkable," but many of the modifying conditions of the molecular activity may certainly be determined, and the remote but necessary influence of these on the mode and intensity of mental action may thus to some extent be recognized. (1879: 373)

A review of G. H. Lewes's *The Study of Psychology* in the same issue made the same point:

It is necessary to adopt a new method of research—to translate the facts of consciousness into terms of another class. . . . The new method follows from the assumption, for long tacitly, though fitfully, made by all, that organic and mental processes are strictly correlated; so that a complete analysis of the one would give an equally complete acquaintance with the other: and then, while some terms of the one series may be beyond our reach, the corresponding members of the other series may be accessible. (Benham 1879: 392)

Another corollary to the doctrine of concomitance was the establishment of the idea of an anatomical substratum that somehow (and the mechanism or bridge proposed varied considerably) "gave rise to" behavior or mind. This was perhaps the most important outcome for the subsequent history of neurophysiology (Angel 1961). As daily work practices subsumed the subtler philosophical questions about the mind/brain connection, they became institutionalized in neurophysiology. Philosophical questions gave way to working assumptions about substrata (see Benham 1880; Ferrier 1880). For example, in Ferrier's *The Functions of the Brain* (1876), he referred to "the anatomical substrata of consciousness" (p. 225) and said: "In order that impressions made on the individual organs of sense shall excite the subjective modification called a sensation, it is necessary that they reach and induce certain molecular changes in the cells of their respective cortical centers" (p. 257).

"Mental operations," or mind, "in the last analysis must be merely the subjective side of sensory and motor substrata" (p. 256); the mechanism of connection between the mind and the brain Ferrier called a "molecular thrill" (p. 258). In a later work, *The Localisation of Cerebral Disease* (1878b), he similarly stated that "the physiology and psychology are but different aspects of the same anatomical substrata, [this] is the conclusion to which all modern research tends" (p. 5). But in this work, it was not a "molecular thrill" but gross pathological processes that were said to be the source of concomitance. This was also true of his lesion experiments, yet the switch in levels of analysis from molecules to lesions was not explicitly discussed.

Similarly, there was disagreement and ambivalence in localizationist writings about the composition of the hypothesized anatomical substratum. Ferrier (and others at times) said that: "The various regions of the cortex are linked together by systems of 'associating fibres,' which furnish an anatomical substratum for the associated action of different regions with each other" (1876: 11; see also Dodds 1877–78 for a review of similar opinions). By comparison, Jackson saw the substratum as electrical in nature:

We have, as anatomists and physiologists, to study not ideas, but the material substrata of ideas (anatomy) and the modes and conditions of energising of these substrata (physiology). Where most would say that the speechless patient has lost the memory of words, I would say that he has lost the anatomical substrata of words. The anatomical substratum of a word is a nervous process for a highly special movement of the articulatory series. That we may have an "idea" of the word, it suffices that the nervous process for it energises; it is not necessary that it energises so strongly that currents reach the articulatory muscles. (1932c: 132)

He went on to say, in a passage vividly illustrating his commitment to attend to physical realms:

How it is that from any degree of energising any kind of arrangement of any sort of matter we have "ideas" of any kind is not a point we are here concerned with. Ours is not a psychological inquiry. It is a physiological investigation, and our methods must be physiological. We have no direct concern with "ideas," but with more or less complex processes for impressions and movements. (1932c: 133)

Here again we have a disclaimer of involvement with "mental" processes, coupled with an untestable mechanism ("energizing") that joins two realms.

By contrast with concomitance theories, building-block theories saw mind or consciousness as more directly emergent from combinations of physical units. Henry Maudsley (1890), for example, articulated this view from a philosopher's point of view. He saw mind as what is left over, or even excreted, after the building blocks of reflexes and learned reflexes combine to form nervous action.

Building-block theories, because they are particulate and modular, had several engineering-like advantages. Units could be distributed over the nervous system in different amounts or densities, thus providing a model for localization of function. These theories also answered in a direct way many of the anomalies of noncorrelation faced by all localizationist experimenters and pathologists.

Those who held building-block theories saw consciousness, or mind, as emerging from the building blocks as "sense datum plus memory" (Ferrier 1876: 44) or, as Gowers put it (1855: 117), as a residue or discharge of memory: "Memory, like other mental actions, has its psychical side. Every functional state of the nerve elements leaves behind it a change in their nutrition, a residual state, in consequence of which the same functional action occurs more readily than before; and this residual disposition is increased by repetition."

Dodds, in a detailed summary of localizationist doctrine (1877–78), exemplified many of the problems faced by localizationists in using a building-block model to solve the problems of parallelism. He also showed how they came to resolve anomalies. Dodds wondered about what explanation could be given of Ferrier's experimental evidence for a functionally differentiated motor region. It is not, he thought, that there is actually a center for the sensory phenomena; instead:

The only probable explanation appears to us to be that the cells of this motor region of Ferrier form, as it were, the motor alphabet of the will. In a way as yet not understood, the will is able to decide upon certain movements, and then, compositor-like, to pick out the area, by whose stimulation the desired result is accomplished. (p. 357)

Dodds's compositor image reflected a concern with the idea of coordination. What coordinated the parts of action? A key passage from Ferrier illustrates the major change in emphasis on this question brought about by the localizationists:

Hence we are not entitled to say that mind, as a unity, has a local inhabitation in any one part of the encephalon, but rather that mental manifestations in their entirety depend on the conjoint action of several parts, the functions of which are capable, within certain limits, of being individually differentiated from each other. (1876: 42)

The problems of the origin and consequence of conjoint action were never fully resolved by localizationist researchers. Instead, the ideas of concomitance and building-block models became themselves increasingly robust because they were useful in addressing clinical issues and in doing experimental work. The problems of storage, coordination, and the mechanism of connection between the two realms were handled by representation theories.

Representation theories were the most philosophically sophisticated of the plausible bridges constructed by localizationists. They were also the most complete in the number and variety of phenomena addressed. They bridged the gap between the mind and body by postulating that activity from one realm was translated across via some sort of algorithm. Indications were made across realms that represented movements, ideas, words, or physiological processes. As Jackson said, "We understand a speaker because he arouses our words" (1932f: 206).

Representation theories arose in part from the observations made in treating the different forms of aphasia. One of the core philosophical problems addressed by representation theories was that of "consciousness versus unconsciousness," or automatic versus reflexive conscious activity. Early on, clinicians were confronted with patients who apparently could think but who could not speak. These patients could intelligently (by gesture) answer questions, showing that they heard and understood words. Yet they were mute. Jackson and other writers analyzed this phenomenon to try to distinguish word understanding and word articulation capacities. This in turn raised the question of whether there was, in Jackson's terms, "inner" and "outer" speech. Were the patients talking to themselves inside their heads? Was this a different "speech" than that which is articulated aloud? These questions would continue to fascinate neurologists for many years (Head 1926; Riese 1977).

Jackson used the concept of representation to resolve these questions in two ways. First, he postulated the existence of inner and outer domains of experience, most notably inner speech and outer (articulated) speech, as well as inner muscle sensations versus outward movements:

A word is a psychical thing, but of course there is a physical process correlative with it. I submit that this physical process is a discharge of cerebral nervous arrangements representing articulatory muscles in a particular movement, or, if there be several syllables, in a series of particular movements. (1932f: 205)

In speaking aloud there is a strong discharge of the same nervous arrangements with a correlative vivid psychical state—in this case the discharge is so strong that lower motor centres are engaged, and finally there are movements of the articulatory muscles in a particular sequence. (1932f: 207)

Second, he mapped evolutionary changes onto the individual, saying that processes of dissolution were ordinally represented, beginning in the larger natural spheres and descending to the individual. These representations could be shown faintly or vividly in the individual nervous system, mere echoes or actual imprints of external events (Walshe 1961). The concept of representation solved some of the contradictions and gaps that remained with the doctrine of concomitance. Specifically, it served to transform static functions into terms more compatible with physiology and to avoid some of the previous philosophical objections to the idea of a substratum. Jackson's definition of anatomy here was unique: "To give an account of the anatomy of any centre is to draw what *parts of the body it represents*, and the ways in which it represents them" (1932d: 96).

Engelhardt (1972) says that Jackson transformed psychological notions of cerebral localization (which he said were outside the province of medicine) into physiological and sensory-motor concepts via the use of the concept of substratum. Jackson then *redefined* anatomy in terms of representation and transformed the physiological concepts into anatomical ones. This, in turn, was tied to parallelist, localized models of the brain.[5] In Jackson's words:

It is an anatomical division. By anatomical I mean that it is after the different degree of complexity, cf., or representation of parts of the body by different centres. The nervous system is a sensorimotor mechanism, a coordinating system from top to bottom. The evolutionist can take a brutally materialistic view of disease of any part of the nervous system, for the reason that he does *not* take a materialistic view of mind—does not confound nervous states with psychical states. The highest centres are only exceedingly complex, and special sensorimotor nervous arrangements representing, or coordinating . . . the whole organism. The doctrine of evolution has nothing whatever to do with the nature of the relation of psychical to the physical states of these centres; it simply affirms concomitance of psychical states with states of these centres. (1932e: 40–41)

Here again Jackson addressed the important audience of evolutionary theorists. Evolutionary biology had long concerned itself with its own species of the mind/brain problem: How did "consciousness," or that which makes humans uniquely human, evolve? Huxley (1904 [1874]) and others had postulated a progression from automatic to reflexive or voluntary activities based on the evolution of the brain. Human beings retained automaton-like movements in the lower part of the nervous system, the animal part. Higher functions were contained in, and localized within, the higher cortical centers. Jackson, drawing on Spencer's ideas of increasing heterogeneity with evolution, saw an increasingly complex, localized human brain as the inevitable outcome of evolutionary processes (1932a, 1932b). His 1884 Croonian lectures to the Royal College of Physicians (1932a) concluded that the highest centers, which make up the "physical basis of consciousness," are the most complex and the most voluntary (although the least organized in the sense that they are naturally ordered). They draw, via representation, on lower centers. An 1873 article of Jackson's had stated that: "Lesions . . . *discharge through* the corpus striatum. I suppose that these convolutions represent over again, but in new and more complex combinations, the very same movements which are represented in the corpus striatum. They are, I believe, the corpus striatum 'raised to a higher power'" (1873a: 200; see also 1932b: 218–19).

In sum, then, representation theories are a kind of Cartesian sign language, where the body and mind mutely gesture across the epistemological gap of parallelism.

Jettisoning Unsolvable "Mind" Problems

It was in part the emphasis on the practical primacy of the physical sphere that made possible the third strategy used by localizationists to explain the contradictions of parallelism: jettisoning unsolvable "mind"-related problems into other lines of work. This division of labor ensured that neurologists and surgeons could concentrate on the physical basis of disease.

The creation of "garbage categories" is a process familiar to medical sociologists. When faced with phenomena that do not fit diagnostic or taxonomic classification schemes, doctors often make residual diagnoses. One function of such diagnoses is to shunt unmanageable, incurable, or undiagnosable patients into other spheres of care where they will not interfere with the ongoing work. Hysteria, senility, and depression, for example, have been criticized as such categories (see Henig 1981).

Localizationists created such categories for problems that did not have an identifiable localized referent or the possibility of a physical treatment. These patients were diagnosed as hysteric or neuraesthenic. In the 1870's and 1880's, patients so diagnosed were treated by the hospital at Queen Square. They received much the same treatments as patients with brain tumors, stroke, or other diseases with known physical referents. By the turn of the century, however, patients diagnosed with "mental" problems—as opposed to physical—began to be referred to psychiatrists and thus to be jettisoned from the jurisdiction of localizationist neurologists and surgeons. This practice both reinforced the physical orientation of these workers and mirrored the philosophy of parallelism on an organizational level. In an active sense, it helped to solve the contradictions posed by parallelism by lodging "mind" and "brain" in the ordinary division of labor and referral system in medicine. (Strauss et al. 1964 analyze a similar phenomenon in contemporary psychiatric institutions.)

SEVEN

The Legacy of Localizationism

> It thus turns out that the old, old dread and dislike of matter as something opposed to mind and threatening it, to be kept within the narrowest bounds of recognition; something to be denied so far as possible lest it encroach upon ideal purposes and finally exclude them from the real world, is as absurd practically as it was impotent intellectually. Judged from the only scientific standpoint, what it does and how it functions, matter means conditions.
>
> —John Dewey (1920: 72)

The legacy of a successful scientific theory is not always found in the validity of its specific findings, but rather in the structure of its axioms and assumptions. The details of Freudian theory have been disputed since its inception, and there are today relatively few orthodox practitioners of Freud's clinical methods. But the long-term impact of the theory is what remains taken for granted: that childhood experience "sets" adult character and that there are unconscious motivations for behavior. Similarly, Darwinian biology created an enduring vision of natural life as a struggle for survival, with scarce resources leading to the diversity of species.

The possibility of "pure" localizationism receded further as the anomaly of inconstant correlation persisted. Yet the legacy of the localizationists is not to be found in a theory that was successful on its own internal terms. Instead, Jackson, Ferrier, Horsley, Gowers, and the other localizationist physician/physiologists framed some basic axioms about the nature of the brain and mind that have persisted to the present day. These subtler assumptions have become deeply entrenched in the institutional structures and work practices of neurophysiology. Such assumptions include the "logic of deletion," which informed the classic localizationist experiments (the idea that function can be studied by removing a physical area); the idea that there is a physical substratum for thought and that the two realms operate in tandem; and the notion that the mind is created of divisible entities with local residences. The legacy also assumes that the mind is contained within the individual and that in some sense the structure of the human brain recapitulates human phylogeny.

These principles continue to be captured not only in ideas about the brain and the mind but also in a set of institutionalized practices and findings. For example, much of neuroanatomy has been based on the search for localized function. The sheer accumulation of data, techniques, and trained personnel in the field has helped to shape the search for function.

Sherrington's Diffusionist Localizationism

The work of Charles Scott Sherrington provided an important bridge between the earlier localizationists and subsequent developments in neurophysiology. Sherrington's *The Integrative Action of the Nervous System* (1906) was dedicated to Ferrier, "in token recognition of his many services to the experimental physiology of the central nervous system." Sherrington described the brain as a labile organ without discrete fixed areas in the strict sense. He emphasized its integrative aspect—the ways in which he saw action as arising from combinations of reflexes and adaptive functions—not, like earlier localizationists, from its modular components or from discrete anatomical pathways (Swazey 1969; Greenblatt 1972).

How could Sherrington's work, seemingly so diffusionist, be hailed as the crowning achievement of localizationism? One important part of the answer is in Sherrington's affirmation of the tacit assumptions of localizationism: parallelism, individualism, idealism, and the hierarchical functional ordering of nervous structure. For example, the following statement from *Integrative Action* echoes Jackson's approach to psychophysical parallelism and recalls Dodds's image of a "compositor of the will" that was articulated in the 1870's and quoted above (p. 170):

It is significant that, although the reflexes controlled are so often unconscious, consciousness is adjunct to the centres which exert the control. . . . Certain it is that if we study the process by which in ourselves this control over reflex action is acquired by an individual, psychical factors loom large, and more is known of them than of the purely physiological *modus operandi* involved in the attainment of the control. . . . It is found that kinaesthetic sensations of the movement to be acquired or controlled, though helpful, are less important than the resident sensations from the part in its "resting" state. (1906: 390)

Sherrington also reaffirmed many of the difficulties with psycho-physical parallelism, but, unlike earlier solutions to the problem, he proposed a new unit of analysis by which to resolve it: the integration of reflexes. He called this a "practical inference" and did not claim that it resolved any philosophical difficulties. Yet his solution was identical with that of Jackson's representation theories, which symbolically communicate across domains:

This practical inference need not in the least involve any doctrinal attitude whatever toward the hypothesis of psycho-physical parallelism. It may proceed quite apart from that. It simply insists on the likeness of nervous reactions expressed by muscular and other effector-organs to reactions whose evidence is sensual. It insists on this likeness being close and fundamental enough to make each of the two classes of phenomena of use to the student of the other. (Sherrington 1906: 396)

Sherrington's exposition of the adaptive functions of the brain, the development of volition, and the integration of reflexes had two important consequences. First, it reaffirmed the assumptions of localizationism, and it did so elegantly and succinctly. Second, it provided a clear resolution to the anomaly of inconstant correlation by declaring it a *discovery* that can be explained by localizationist theory. If actions must be synthesized, or even averaged, across numbers of centers, then the idea of a one-to-one correlation between part and function makes no sense. Yet, and this is crucial, the central idea of correlation of anatomy and function is preserved and *all the evidentiary, clinical, and institutional infrastructures built up by localizationists remain intact*.

It was important that Sherrington's exposition, however diffusionist, not violate institutionalized work practices. Andrew Peacock argues that:

"Busy commonsense" had been a very useful approach in both the 19th and 20th centuries. Knowledge of neurophysiology had been greatly advanced by the analytic approach to biological phenomena: The traditional line of demarcation between mind and body had been pushed further and further back, and there was no longer much dispute that there were discrete areas of the brain representing "lower" motor and sensory functions. For the "higher" functions, there was no such agreement. Here the "localizationists" believed that all "higher" functions would eventually be localized, while the "holists" maintained that such functions were the product only of the integral brain. Thus, both parties agreed that a structure-function relationship existed; they were only disagreed about the interpretation of this relationship. (1982: 92)

The interpretation of the relationship was to undergo several more transmogrifications in the decades following Sherrington, all of which attested to the remarkable strength of the localizationist perspective.

From Sherrington to Contemporary Neurophysiology

World War I drastically changed the status and resources of neurological surgery. This period saw the advent of new forms of weaponry; a hitherto unimaginable number of soldiers were involved in battle; and for the first time medical doctors and surgeons worked together with virtually unlimited numbers of cases involving brain injuries. Head wounds, battle shock, and mental disorders resulting from trauma occurred on a hitherto unknown scale (Horrax 1952; Sachs 1952).

Sherrington's subtle physiological model did not fill the desperate need for simple, quick, and effective diagnostic procedures that could correlate an injury with a loss of function. On the battlefield or in the neuropsychiatric hospital, it was difficult to use such a subtle theory to locate a site for rough-and-ready emergency surgery or bullet removal (United States Surgeon-General's Office 1919; Cushing 1935; McGill University 1936). In light of thousands of battle casualties and head wounds, a simpler location/function model was again invoked in medicine and in the new field of neuropsychiatry. Sherrington's "discovery" appeared somewhat tangential to practicing clinicians and those developing neuropsychiatric taxonomies. As such, however, it did not interfere with clinical and research programs based on one-to-one models of the relationship between area and function.

By the end of the war, an enormous volume of data had been collected on head wounds, shock, and trauma. The data were slowly sorted through. Professional associations that were formed during the war obtained funding and increased legitimacy (Cushing 1920). Much of the data so collected was interpreted by another group in the brain research arena: psychologists and psychiatrists. An important alliance was formed at this time between neurosurgeons and psychiatrists, reflected in the emergence of the term "neuropsychiatry" (Star 1982). Partly because of the large number of mentally injured soldiers, there was an enormous demand for psychiatrists to treat veterans. Neuropsychiatry as a full-fledged field quickly established itself.

The alliance was an important one, similar to the earlier meshing of resources by neurology and surgery. Psychiatrists were able to provide explanations for supposedly nonphysical phenomena, and neurosurgeons provided physical techniques for organic problems. Together, the two specialties claimed to explain almost all behavioral and perceptual problems (Merritt 1975), and again there was an instantiation of the mind/brain division of labor.

By the 1930's specialized neurosurgical and neuropsychiatric institutions had developed, such as the Montreal Neurological Institute (McGill University 1936). Training in the specialty was instituted in most medical schools. In all of these research programs the localizationist perspective continued to prevail, sometimes in its tacit form and sometimes explicitly.

Explicit localizationism reached its apex in the 1940's and 1950's with the rise of psychosurgery and the work of Wilder Penfield and Lamar Roberts (Peacock 1982). They used a localizationist approach to specify regions thought responsible for memory, epilepsy, and parts of the personality. A famous photograph of an operation by Penfield shows an exposed brain covered with tiny numbered slips of paper; these slips represent the different functions thought to be located in each area. Ferrier's enterprise was thus transferred directly to the living brain and incorporated into clinical practice (Penfield and Roberts 1959). (Compare Figures 2 and 3, which show an early diagram of Ferrier's and the photograph from Penfield's brain surgery, respectively.) The psychosurgery programs of that period sought to remove the sites of "aggression" and antisocial behavior (Vaughan 1975).

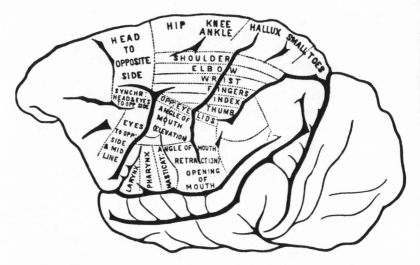

Fig. 2. Motor areas according to Beevor and Horsley, in Ferrier 1890: 32. These areas were localized by applying electrical current to the surface of the brain. Both animal and human data seem to have been integrated here by Ferrier.

In all of this work we can see the persistent conception of a physical "substratum" carrying mental function; of approaches based on a logic of deletion; and of the divisible, particulate, and individual mind.

Modern Neurophysiology: Regions, Substrata, and the Division of Labor

The amount of neurophysiological research on brain and nervous system function has geometrically increased since Sherrington's time, in terms of resources, numbers of lines of work and problems involved, and the impact on other lines of scientific inquiry. As the field has grown, new lines of work have become involved that did not develop historically from institutions based on localizationism. The disciplines involved range from rehabilitation medicine and biochemistry to computer science and physics.

A fascinating situation thus exists in the present-day "neurosciences." Older disciplines with epistemological bases in localization-

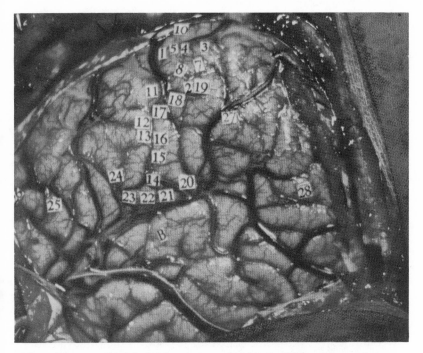

Fig. 3. Photograph of the left hemisphere of C. H., Penfield's seizure patient. During surgery, Penfield performed experiments on his patients. The numbers on the surface of the cortex indicate locations where electrical current was applied to the cortex. Patients were required to talk, write, count, and read during the electrical stimulation (patients are conscious during brain surgery, since the brain itself cannot sense pain). Responses were then analyzed in order to map the speech areas of the brain. (Use of the photograph from Penfield and Roberts 1959 by permission of the publisher.)

ism are incorporating results from outsiders who do not share those assumptions. Often, this incorporation is in the form of technologies; for example, the development of the PET-scan (positron emission tomography, a method for scanning brain activity using radioactive injected substances) represents the intersection of nuclear physics and localizationist neurology. The nature and kinds of debate about cognition and consciousness that have arisen in recent years reflect the persistent legacy of localizationism.

It is clearly beyond the scope of a chapter or book of this nature to review modern neurosciences. Let me restrict my comments to several ways in which I perceive the localizationist legacy to be influencing modern neurophysiology.

In reading modern neurosciences with an eye to the localizationist influence, one becomes quickly aware of three strains. First, the search for localized regions tied to specific functions continues to occupy many researchers. Second, there is a continued search for a substratum of mind, using anatomical/physiological techniques. Much of the search is based on and enhanced by new techniques for studying the brain: the PET-scan, various injections, and new imaging technology. Third, the division of labor between "mind" lines of work and "brain" lines of work continues to be strongly represented. This can be seen most recently, and in its most popular form, in the rise of "connectionism" (also called parallel distributed processing) and its relation to "brain" lines of work.

The Search for Localized Regions

Contemporary neurophysiological literature often takes for granted many of the regions defined by early localizationists while it continues to redefine the search for regions. In the latter case, this means arguments about the nature of localization: is it based on topography, cortical layers, symbolic representation, habit, evolution, or genetics? Joaquin Fuster (1980), for example, reviews work on the frontal cortex and attempts to localize disorders of affect, emotion and cognition, the sense of temporal order, and human evolution. He states:

A wealth of experimental evidence now indicates that the functions of the prefrontal cortex are essentially few in number, that they are represented over the cortical surface according to a certain topological pattern, and, most important, that they are interrelated, mutually supporting and complementing each other in the purposive behavior of the organism. (p. 1)

Localization of regions has been a compelling concern in clinical practice, especially (still) with chronically ill populations such as epileptics and people with brain injuries or learning disabilities. Many scholars explicitly acknowledge the impact of the early localizationists on their work (such as Thompson and Green 1982). For example, Theodore Rasmussen says:

Since the days of Hughlings Jackson a hundred years ago, localization of epileptic seizures and epileptic mechanisms has been mainly concerned with the site of origin of the epileptic disturbance responsible for the clinical epileptic seizure. This continues to be of primary importance for physicians responsible for treating patients with epilepsy. (1982: 177)

And Sandra Witelson states:

Functional differentiation of the cerebral cortex clearly exists. The localization of different cognitive functions in the anteroposterior plane of the human brain, first noted in the nineteenth century and exemplified by the different functions of the frontal and posterior language regions, has been easy to conceptualize in anatomical terms. (1983: 117)

The idea that there are specialized functions in the right and left hemispheres has been a major concern of modern neurophysiology. In sheer numbers, it is perhaps the most compelling contemporary legacy of localizationism: the search for specialized functions in a particular place in the brain. There are thousands of articles, scholarly and popular, on the right-brain/left-brain concept (see, for example, Kinsbourne 1978; Witelson 1983). Again, the topics covered are numerous. For example, a volume edited by Alfredo Ardila and Feggy Ostrosky-Solis (1984) covers the right hemisphere's function in behavior, evolution, language, emotions, aphasia, development, bilingualism, and lesion effects in rats. Similarly, Andrew Young (1983) details many attempts to find differences in function in cerebral asymmetry; Joseph LeDoux, in an article in the Young volume, states:

A potpourri of psychological phenomena, from poetic inspiration to joggers' high, from scientific creativity to sexual orgasm and more, have been conveniently explained with the now familiar retort: 'It's a . . . hemisphere function.' The mind is not easily dichotomised in a way that provides much in the way of detailed insight into psychological processes, and it is naïve to think that the brain is any simpler. No one cognitive function is completely dependent on one hemisphere or another. Complex psychological processes reflect the functioning of both sides of the brain at all levels of the neuraxis, and a theory of how these processes relate to brain mechanisms must account for the integrated functioning of the nervous system." (1983: 212)

This quote indicates simultaneously a rejection of "strict" localization of function and an acceptance of the idea of regions and of substrata.

Modern neurophysiologists often find that many of the epistemological and philosophical questions that preoccupied nineteenth-century neurologists remain structurally similar. Witelson has addressed the unresolved issues of individual differences and the degree of laterality (the degree of right/left differentiation):

> Does 'bihemispheric' representation involve duplicated representation of a cognitive function in both hemispheres (a 'twin' situation), or does it involve a divided representation of a cognitive function with some aspects lateralized to one hemisphere and other aspects within the same general mode represented in the other hemisphere (a 'subdivision of labor' situation)? (1983:120)

This directly echoes the concerns of Jackson, Brown-Séquard, and Horsley as detailed earlier in this volume: Where are the functions located? Are they divisible? If so, how can we know it?

Modern Work on the Substrata

The idea that there is a substratum of matter that carries mind upon it was created in modern form by the nineteenth-century localizationists, as we have seen. This link between localization and the concept of substrata arises logically: if you are looking for a function "residing" in one particular place, the work divides into finding the place and linking it with the function. In modern neurophysiology, this idea still has a great deal of purchase. The focus for many contemporary neurophysiologists seems to be on a continuation of the search for what may underlie localized phenomena, using a new, more sophisticated array of tools and technologies with which to probe the tissues of the brain (see, for example, Raichler 1982 on positron emission tomography; McEachron 1986 on computer-assisted autoradiography).

Norman Geschwind and Albert Galaburda (1987) make a strong argument for a structural substratum for behavior on the basis of asymmetrical anatomical variations. They state that this variation may begin with the actual physical structure of matter and that it may have ramifications at the behavioral and social level as well. They look for anomalies in structure and seek to correlate them with anomalies in function. A volume edited by Andrew Kertesz (1983) reviews many of the structure/function issues from the point of view of neuropsychology. The contents are strikingly similar in terms of basic assumptions to much earlier work: lesion size and lesion locus in aphasia, localization of language and vision by electrical stimulation, localization of lesions in Broca's motor aphasia, frontal lobe lesions and behavior, and so on.

The Mind / Brain Division of Labor

Neuroscientists realize that, by the strict rules of inference and causality ideally exemplified by the scientific method, they are still on shaky philosophical ground in discussions of the brain and mind. Yet there is an ongoing debate in and around modern neuroscience about the nature of the mind/brain relationship (see Popper and Eccles 1977; Edelman and Mountcastle 1978; Schmitt and Worden 1979; Reichardt and Poggio 1981), and this relationship is the focus of numerous review papers and articles debating aspects of the philosophical foundations (see MacKay 1978; Sperry 1980). The terms of the debate have not changed significantly since the late nineteenth century, with one apparent exception: the introduction of computer terminology into the discussion of brain modeling. Although Huxley and others discussed automata theory in the light of various biological and neurological theories at that time, it was not until World War II that the terminology of computation and computers came to dominate one large sector of discussion about the mind and the brain.

The basic question involves two points, both of which are rooted in localizationism: (1) Is there a division between brain (the material organ) and mind (perception, "thought," or behavior)? (2) If there is such a division, what is its nature? Does brain "produce" mind or does mind produce brain functions to suit its needs? Positions on this fundamental question range from those approaches that emphasize *brain* to the exclusion of *mind* ("radical materialist") to those that reverse the emphasis ("disembodied idealist"). Participants in the mind/ brain debate include philosophers, physicians, neuroscientists, and a substantial number of outsiders, including journalists and theologians. Professional journals, meetings, and interest groups have formed around the debate. As in Ferrier's day, neuroscientists are aware of philosophical problems with parallelism and often agree with criticisms of their own work.

Yet, as in the nineteenth century, a division of labor remains between "mind" and "brain," a division that is for the most part unexamined in the philosophical discourse. Most recently, this division appears between cognitive science and neuroscience.

Alongside the neurophysiologists and anatomists concerned with probing structure, laterality, and differential anatomy, a powerful group of cognitive scientists is allied both with neurosciences and with computer sciences. One subgroup of cognitive scientists, known as the "connectionists," perhaps best illustrates one part of the legacy of the division of labor along mind/brain lines. (Connectionists work on a set of problems they call "parallel distributed processing," or PDP [Rumelhart, McClelland, and the PDP Research Group 1986; McClelland, Rumelhart, and the PDP Research Group 1986].)

Connectionism is a new approach to models of mind and cognition, or to representation. It is an abstract theory, in principle applicable to any phenomenon, describing the ways in which very simple actions may be combined to create more complex ones, including representations of actions.

The relationship between connectionist models and brain function is a source of concern to connectionists themselves. The primary argument of the PDP group volumes is that connectionism may model basic computational processes and basic cognitive processes. The relationship to actual brain functioning is assumed and/or approximated:

One reason for the appeal of PDP models is their obvious "physiological flavor." They seem so much more closely tied to the physiology of the brain than are other kinds of information processing models. The brain consists of a large number of highly interconnected elements which apparently send very simple excitatory and inhibitory messages to each other. (McClelland, Rumelhart, and Hinton 1986:10)

David Rumelhart and James McClelland also state that:

We believe that an understanding of the relationships between cognitive phenomena and brain functions will evolve slowly. We also believe that cognitive theories can provide a useful source of information for the neuroscientist. We do not, however, believe that current knowledge from neuroscience provides no guidance to those interested in the functioning of the mind. We have not, by and large, focused on the kinds of constraints which arise from detailed analysis of particular circuitry and organs of the brain. Rather we have found that information concerning brain-style processing has itself been very provocative in our model building efforts. (1986: 130)

Terrence Sejnowski echoes this sentiment with a statement that, although neuroscientists "may feel uncomfortable because connectionist models do not take into account much of the known cellular properties of neurons," they may be useful approximations of information processing (1986: 388).

The idea of substrata is important in the connectionist model, and the division of labor implied by the quotes above is clear. In answer to the question of why people are smarter than rats if there is a universal processing "language" such as connectionism, Rumelhart and McClelland state that it is because "People have much more cortex than rats do or even than other primates do; . . . presumably this extra cortex is strategically placed in the brain to subserve just those functions that differentiate people from rats or even apes" (p. 143).

To summarize the contemporary legacy of localizationism: the search for areas remains strong, as does the idea of substrata. Even in a relatively diffusionist theory such as connectionism, this latter idea is reinforced by a mind/brain division of labor across lines of work. This is also true in clinical work, where the need for swift diagnosis may still outweigh subtler or more experimental physiological models.

Science and Work

I have made the argument in this volume that the truth of a theory does not rest upon its match with logical formulations but derives from historical, work-based, and institutional processes within lines of work. This is true for working scientists as well as for sociologists of science "standing outside." (It is also no less true for the sociology and history of science itself.) But scientists are normatively compelled to evaluate their work according to logical ideals.

Thus, as neuroscientists face localization-related logical inconsistencies in their work, there is a constant spate of reform articles and reform movements within the field to try to bring logic in line with practice. This is an attempt to be consistent and honest on the part of neuroscientists. Yet because the grounds for the persistence of the localizationist perspective are not understood in the field and have never been institutionally challenged, criticisms of logical inconsistencies are not effectively rooted in practice.

The persistence of the localizationist perspective is reflected in the very terminology of the debates discussed here. Neuroscientists have discovered that declaring the brain and the mind to be the same thing does not solve the problem. The institutional structures that have separated them are too entrenched, and many of the technologies they use reify and reaffirm psychophysical parallelism. Pulling together multiple levels of analysis in a single project does not challenge the segmentation of fields nor the view of the mind as hierarchical and made of incrementally assembled parts. Attempts to address the anomalies and problems of correlation and causality that do not address the institutional issues cannot be structurally effective.

The growth and entrenchment of the axioms of the localizationist perspective are found in the work practices of localizationists, from the daily work to the institutional fates examined in this book. The structure of that practice meant forming, in Fujimura's terms (1987), "doable" problems from a confusing and disordered open system of events, actors, and negotiations.

Recent work in the sociology of science has indicated that there is an enormous variety in the methods used and conditions under which the complexity of nature gets made simpler and more manageable. Sometimes local politics decide how the field of investigation will be limited. At other times, a narrow focus on one "building block," seen as part of a larger theoretical whole, effectively screens out other complexities. Or the availability of a given piece of machinery will constrain the complexity of the problem. Without X-ray crystallography, for instance, it is difficult to perceive the complex form of the double helix. There is constant reconciling between theoretical commitments and constraints on material resources.

Philosophers of science and many historians have focused almost exclusively on the development of theoretical commitments in science, omitting mention of material constraints. By contrast, many sociologists and economists have often focused exclusively on those material aspects constraining scientific development. From either perspective, the reconciling process per se may remain unexamined.

Scientists themselves lose sight of their reconciliation work, both in execution and in description. Scientific work is complicated: any set of scientific tasks involves multiple problems, qualifications, exigencies, demands, and audiences. To work without getting lost in endless contingencies, scientists must draw boundaries and exclude some kinds of artifacts and complications from consideration. In other words, part of doing science is transforming problems with many contingencies into those simple enough to work on. In "The Structure of Ill-Structured Problems" (1973), Simon discusses this transformation. He notes that computer scientists ordinarily distinguish between "well-structured" and "ill-structured" problems. Well-structured problems are those for which all possible contingencies can be programmed—no new contingencies arise as a result of the problem-solving process. Ill-structured problems, on the other hand, develop new and unpredictable contingencies in the course of solution.

In fact, the number of significant, well-structured problems in the real world is almost nil. Scientists break ill-structured problems into pieces that they work on *as if* they were well-structured, in order to get the work done. Creating well-structured problems requires ignoring complexity: uncertainties in the environment, subjects' or patients' reactions, unforeseen interaction effects. In order to actually do the research, lines and boundaries must be drawn around complications, implications, and exceptions. Goals, images, and tasks simple enough to manage are developed. Simon (1973) notes that in the process of transforming ill-structured problems into well-structured ones, the relationships between well-structured problems are ignored. Learning to manage all of the difficulties that arise from these relationships is a major part of professional training and "maturity."

The process of creating well-structured problems from ill-structured ones is an essential part of scientific work. However, in conjunction with the deletion of descriptions of this process from scientists' descriptions of their work, scientific "facts" become reified and their production histories lost. Those histories are further obscured by the shorthand of formal professional modes of presenting results that are typically both brief and idiosyncratic within lines of

work. Retrieving those histories, by observing the process of deletion, provides us with important data about the connection between
work process and theories (Fleck 1979 [1935]; Latour and Woolgar
1979; Latour 1980; Woolgar 1981; Callon, Law, and Rip 1986).

Sociologists of science have begun to investigate some aspects of
the "social construction" of scientific reality. Much of this work has
focused on the deletion of detail that occurs at the publication and
analysis stages. For example, Latour and Woolgar developed a scale
of measurement of reification of facts. This scale measured how scientists remove actions from written presentations ("deletion of modalities"). As others have noted (Collins 1975; Barnes and Law 1976),
published scientific conclusions do not represent all details of the
work scientists perform. Instead, results present partial or schematic
maps of the original work. These maps emphasize ideal or logical developments. They may form the basis for further research in other
work sites, because other labs use them to help shape their ongoing
work. But scientists also make the tacit assumption that scientific facts
are fully detailed representations of the work—thus that they are fully
detailed maps. As many have demonstrated (Dewey and Bentley 1949;
Stanley and Robbins 1977; Garfinkel, Lynch, and Livingston 1981),
the stylistic canons of scientific writing require that results be presented as *faits accomplis* without mention of production or decision-
making processes.

Another aspect of the deletion of work descriptions has been explored by Harry Collins and Trevor Pinch (1982). They begin with
the observation that there is no such thing as a fully detailed rendition
of scientific work. Variation and discretion are always present in the
scientific work site, and complete replication is a chimera. Something
differs in every experimental replication. Collins and Pinch examine
the conditions under which scientists invoke this variability as a problem or under which they apply more rigid rules for replication.

Mechanisms for scientific review of the gap between work processes and work representations (publications) are informal and often
unspecified. Thus, by manipulating the rules of replication, scientists
can make legitimate and illegitimate designations about research.
Collins and Pinch use the example of ESP (extrasensory perception)
research and its career in trying to become legitimate. Main-line researchers have demanded that ESP experiments be replicated accord-

ing to much more stringent standards than those upheld in "normal" science-making. When ESP researchers are unable to replicate, this is taken as disproving the existence of ESP. Brian Wynne (1979) has documented a similar case from a historical perspective. Michael Lynch (1982) has also discussed the lack of specification and the re-creation of diagnostic categories in the clinical testing situation. In his research, the rules were manipulated according to the social status of the patients as well as the research needs of doctors.

This work in the sociology of science points to a wide, informal zone where bargaining takes place about how well structured problems must be. This wide negotiation zone spans many stages of work, from research design to publication. There is ample room at any stage to lose sight of the process of transformation from ill-structured to well-structured problem. John Law's work (1986) shows that the scope of this zone may be wider than the discipline itself, because actors "black-box" the complexities of one another's results—that is, they take what is apparent on the surface and trust that the rest is coherently there, ignoring content. We saw a similar process in clinical/basic triangulation of localizationist work in Chapter 4. Edward Manier's analysis (1986) of interfield communication in neurophysiology provides a provocative contemporary example of this.

The fitting process between theoretical commitments and the constraints on material resources can be examined on a number of organizational levels. Large-scale debates or historical change in scientific perspectives result in changed methods, technologies, and problems. These large-scale changes can also result in professional movements and changed institutional configurations (Busch 1982). On a smaller organizational scale, individual laboratories or research programs can be studied to reveal how they "fit" theories with constraints. Similarly, scientists' representations of their work can be studied at many stages, from selection of problems to organization of project to final publication.

This book presented a working example of the development of a successful scientific theory, examining the fitting between materials, organizations, and theories at several levels of organization. Localizationists, in essence, built an anomaly-devouring machine, a way of looking at the brain and the mind that became extraordinarily robust—that is, both plastic and coherent. Several aspects of the theory's development from an open system were intertwined through different contexts of work: inertia, momentum, incompleteness at any one point, cumulative reification and generative entrenchment, and progressive inseparability of parts. Through the expression of these aspects in the localizationist enterprise, the open system of the scientific workplace gave birth to a robust theory. In concluding, I will review the ways in which these dimensions were significant in the various situations discussed in the chapters above.

Inertia

The theory of localization of function was linked with medical reforms and became an important selling point for research. As part of the professionalization process, doctors began to try to reserve evaluation of clinical results to the medical profession. Professional change contributed to inertia through this privatizing of evaluation. Once instituted, results became difficult to challenge from the outside and were linked with the legitimacy of medicine itself.

The combination and substitution of different domains of evidence meant that the legitimation of the theory and routine problems of implementation were entangled. Once established, these approaches were difficult to dismantle because of their bases in multiple and shifting work and evidentiary domains. Also, the triangulation of evidence merged problems from multiple sites. Such solutions became difficult to challenge.

The strong link between clinical taxonomies and clinical programs contributed to the inertial properties of the theory. The slow accumulation of cases to support localizationist arguments entrenched them in canonical medical journals and training programs. By gradually collecting examples, localizationists created an inert pile of evidence that became difficult to move.

Momentum

The alliance between the development of the theory of localization and medical reformers contributed to its momentum. Common legitimation sped up adoption of the theory in different sites. The rising status of physicians and surgeons meant that the theory was picked up and used by many rapidly growing groups. The standard diagnostic categories developed by localizationists could quickly be adopted by multiple lines of work, and the development of universal, standard atlases of the brain made localization models portable and thus easily diffused across sites.

The conduct of the localizationist debate contributed to the theory's momentum. The public demonstrations such as that orchestrated at the 1881 International Medical Congress contributed to momentum through "advertising" and well-staged controversy. Support from evolutionary biology, the promise of genuinely new results for the old arena of debate about the mind and body, and the promise of a working algorithm to map the coincidence of mind and brain phenomena also contributed to momentum by raising expectations about the theory. Although philosophers argued with the parallelism adopted by localizationists, they also picked up and discussed the results of localizationist experiments and helped to spread such results rapidly.

Incompleteness at Any One Point

The momentum of the theory, professional developments, turf battles between specialists and general practitioners, and the rise of specialty hospitals with their separate domains of expertise made the theory impossible to comprehend from any single point. Moreover, anomalies were shuffled between lines of work, often jettisoned from each according to the exigencies of daily work and uncertainty. The partial assimilation and transformation of diffusionist arguments, and the confounding of different aspects of the debate, made arguments slippery and complex, with unclear boundaries around positions.

Reification and Entrenchment

The need for clear, marketable results in medical research meant that theories had to be developed that were easily described, were not terribly complex, and would remain fixed. The movement toward standardized and idealized taxonomies also contributed to reification. This was partly due to the increasing need for standardized hospital training and other similar shifts in medical education.

The dynamics of the debate with diffusionists helped cumulatively to reify the theory by obscuring contradictions and procedural and methodological subtleties. The oversimplified "cartooning" of each side by the other was also a reification.

The use of unprovable categories and the transformation of physiological processes into anatomical distinctions reified many aspects of behavior. In a more subtle way, as parallelism was adopted, the processual and discovered aspects of behavior became transformed into the static correlates of either mind or body. These, in turn, became entrenched in practice.

Inseparability of Parts

Because localizationists were banded together against a common enemy, political alliances forced intellectual alliances and logically necessary connections between vivisection and localization and between evolutionary biology and localization. The institutional base of physiology in medicine and the overlapping social worlds investigating localization also meant that different aspects of localizationism became increasingly intertwined.

Overlapping evidence from different realms made apparently logical connections from originally unconnected points. The hierarchical organization of the nervous system, for example, which was originally derived from evolutionary biology and imported through neurology, became linked to the idea of a nervous substratum. This was strengthened by pathological evidence and surgical approaches.

Methods of argument can establish taxonomies and help to redefine anomalies. Certain questions become salient, others are derided. Debating tactics in the localizationist debate confounded the grounds for evaluating obduracy and robustness, because *ad hominem* tactics, demonstrations, cross-legitimation, and various forms of diplomacy were commingled by those on different sides of the debate.

The conflation of different aspects of the debate (such as vivisection with the validity of localization; see Chapter 2) helped to make the parts of the localizationist perspective progressively more difficult to separate. In addition, using the unknown to extend the perspective into future or untestable realms often resulted in creating necessary "logical" connections between parts of the theory, which were later legitimated.

The philosophical difficulties with parallelism arise as boundaries from different work realms are assumed to coincide. Material and immaterial evidence is assumed to be coincident. Localizationism became more obdurate as this mixture of material and immaterial, concrete and abstract categories became a tacit part of research. As phenomena that localizationists saw as material and as immaterial were presumed to have coincident boundaries, parts of the perspective became inseparable.

The localization theory changed in several respects as it developed from 1870 to 1906. The tacit and explicit parts of the theory became more tightly articulated during the course of its development. In 1870, localizationist researchers had an organizing schema of the brain and nervous system but little data to verify it. This was true in two respects: they had little data to verify the overall view of the brain as divided into areas, and they had little data then to assign areas on the basis of function. Similarly, they had no clinical proof that localization theory would be helpful for treating patients. Localizationists at that time were working, clinically, with an extremely unclear taxonomic scheme (classification of diseases) and a poorly developed set of diagnostic tools. In England, links to physiology from clinical medicine were mostly speculative. Physiology was a physician's hobby whose value was not universally acknowledged.

By 1906 many of these conditions had changed dramatically. Over the 36 years examined here, the main direction of effort was overwhelmingly addressed not to the problem of *whether* the brain could be divided into areas but *which* areas could be located where. By concentrating on such areas, researchers often sidestepped the question of whether there were areas at all. They achieved striking success in comparison with their earlier situation. They were able to link localization theory with several clinical treatments, including that for epilepsy and, especially, for brain surgery. They clarified taxonomic and diagnostic uncertainties on the basis of localization theory, and they made alliances with professional physiologists (such as Sharpey-Schafer and Foster) and evolutionary biologists (including Darwin and Huxley). They explicitly linked their programs of physiological research with the clinical phenomena being addressed by localizationist clinical medicine.

As this book illustrates, localizationists were able to construct a theory in which all of these elements were strongly linked. The picture of the brain and nervous system that emerged at the end of the period was that the nervous system was constructed in an evolutionary hierarchy which could be investigated through disease or experiment (see, for example, Brunton 1882). Diseases were seen as experiments made by nature (Jackson 1873a) and could therefore provide basic information about the composition of the nervous system. Breakdowns in behavioral function were believed to have an anatomical base. The localizationist researchers at Queen Square had done the exemplary experiments on localization of function, and they were experts at treating related diseases.

We can see that localizationists eventually intertwined questions about the nature of phenomena, the strategies for organizing information and resources, and political commitments.

The Implications of Analyzing Science as Work

Research on scientific theories has rarely taken into account the processes and dimensions described above, especially the degree to which these complex multiple dimensions are interactive and developmental. What are the implications for looking at theories in this way? A conversation with Anselm Strauss provided a partial answer to this question. As I was describing to him the many participants in the debate about localization, and the various kinds of work and uncertainties faced by participants, I began to frame the concept "inertia." I saw the questions becoming extraordinarily complex and, at the same time, taken for granted by participants. In the middle of explaining this, and when I was feeling overwhelmed with the complexity and interdependence of all the issues, Strauss asked me: what would it have taken to overthrow the theory?

Two very different answers can be given for the beginning and the end of the period examined. In 1870 a funded, well-organized counterprogram with both clinical and basic physiological bases might well have defeated the localizationists in Western Europe (see Todes 1981 for an example of this in Russia). By 1906, however, the perspective was so entrenched that overthrowing it would have taken something more nearly catastrophic. No counterprogram could have found a strong institutional base because no need for it was perceived by either patients or other doctors; counterevidence had already been produced in many other sites and had often been partially assimilated into localizationism.

Understanding the processes and conditions under which such "obvious" and powerful theories about nature take hold is important in several respects. First, such theories about nature have enormous political implications. This has been well documented in the case of racist and sexist theories (see Gould 1981; Hubbard and Lowe 1979), where bias consists of inaccurately characterizing or excluding certain human groups. Less well documented are the political implications of theories without such direct connections. Quantifying, numbering, and localizing, for example, are activities with important consequences for the kinds of choices available to people. In order to understand the issues in any policy decision, these elements need to be examined and understood. They have political ramifications that are often not thought of as political.

Second, the kind of theory/work links sketched here are useful for researching the history of scientific disciplines. Rather than studying simply the diffusion of ideas or the intellectual history of a discipline without its constraining material base, the analysis of work organization provides a new way to look at issues that traditionally have been characterized as *either* "internalist" (solely the ideas and techniques employed by members of the discipline) *or* "externalist" (solely shaped by institutions and politics outside the workplace). The debate about internalist versus externalist history of science has been a long and acrimonious one, parallel in many ways to the "macro"/"micro" debate in sociology. From the analysis of theories presented here, we can see that such distinctions are spurious and that the relationship is dialectical and emergent, not parallel and additive.[1] Problems arise in the course of work owing to the location of and constraints on it. The solution to these problems may change both the way the work is done and the institutional forms within which it is done.

Third, the study of how theories take hold and become seen as "natural" is important in answering some basic questions in the sociology of knowledge and epistemology. This book argues that problems/theories/facts/perspectives are a form of collective behavior, and I have provided some data about the processes and conditions of that behavior. Implicit in this approach is an equation between *knowing* and *working*. These two kinds of events do not proceed in parallel: they are the same activity, but differently reported.

Appendixes

The following appendixes represent diffusionist writings that have been previously unavailable in English. Localizationist writings are more widely available in the English-language medical literature, as referenced. Appendix A is from Goltz, "Discussion on the Localization of Functions in the Cortex Cerebri," in MacCormac 1881 (vol. 1, pp. 218–37) and was translated from the German by Sigrid Novikoff in October 1982. Appendix B is from Panizza 1887 (pp. 148–67) and was translated from the Italian by Mirto Stone in 1982.

Appendix A: Goltz

Morning Session

If we set ourselves the task of investigating the functions of a nervous organ, there are two research methods at our disposal, the stimulation method and the extirpation method. The former seemed to let us down altogether with regard to the research on the functions of the cerebrum; for the older authors admitted unanimously that a stimulation of the exposed surface of the cerebrum produced no results at all. Fritsch and Hitzig proved that this conception nevertheless rests upon an error. They found that, upon electrical stimulation of certain points of the parietal lobe of the dog, convulsive movements occurred in specific muscle groups of the opposite side of the body. Stimulation of a certain spot in the brain causes movements of the front legs, of another spot movement of the hind legs, of the facial muscles, etc. The section of the cerebrum that contains the stimulation points is called the sensitive (excitable) zone or actually the motor zone. But there are also large areas of the brain surface, the stimulation of which remains without reaction, one of which is the occipital lobe (*Hinterlappen*).

The fact that the result of the stimulation is so extremely different, depending on the location of the stimulated point, suggested that the different sections of the cerebrum could be equally different in their functional meaning. But Fritsch and Hitzig also realized that the stimulation method alone would be insufficient to successfully pursue this idea any further. If we see a group of muscles—for example the muscles of the foot—twitch as a result of a stimulation, the nervous system stimulated can be of very different importance.

Whether we stimulate the motor nerves, the spinal cord, the brain, or certain sense nerves, in all cases twitches of the foot muscles can be caused. Therefore, I cannot deduce with certainty from the twitching foot muscle caused by the stimulation of a section of the nervous system what the functional importance of the stimulated organ is. . . .

Therefore all scientists agree that the extirpation method has to complement the stimulation method in order to test it. I hope that many will agree with me when I maintain that the extirpation method is to be preferred because it induces a smaller number of false conclusions.

Fritsch and Hitzig immediately made some extirpation tests. They found that, upon removing that part of the cerebral cortex the stimulation of which had caused twitches in the opposite-side front leg, strange disturbances in the movement of the same limbs occurred, which they interpreted as a result of the loss of the muscle-consciousness. Later Hitzig observed blindness of the opposite-side eye after removal of a piece of the occipital lobe. Fritsch and Hitzig considered these experiences to be sufficient for the establishment of a hypothesis that constitutes a crass opposition to the teaching of Flourens, which had been generally recognized to that date. Flourens taught that all sections of the cerebrum served the same functions. Fritsch and Hitzig believed it to be proven that the cerebral cortex is to be divided into definable individual areas or centers, each of which heads a special function. The investigations of Fritsch and Hitzig were continued, first by Ferrier and then by a number of other scientists. . . . The hypotheses of all these scientists have in common that they divide the cerebral cortex into small defined fields, centers, or spheres and assign special functions to each of them. The most striking differences exist, however, in the spatial delineation and arrangement of the fields and the distribution of the individual functions assigned to them, especially between Ferrier and Munk.

Unconcerned by these contradictions, the medical public accepted these modern localization theories with great applause. A number of textbooks were enthusiastic about them, although one should have hesitated to accuse such a clear mind as Flourens's of such serious mistakes in his observations. The new theories were obviously so trustingly accepted because the ground was prepared for them, as, on the basis of pathological observations, the need for a spatial division of the functions of the cerebrum was felt. The delicate rounding-off of the new theories, the apparent excellent agreement between the stimulation and extirpation methods, had a seductive effect. But a fruit may look very enticing and yet be worm-eaten in its core, and it is not difficult to identify the worm-eaten point in all the localization doctrines mentioned so far. It is the ways and means by which the various authors handle themselves with respect to the so-called restitution question. Hitzig, Ferrier, and all their successors admit that the disturbances that occur after the extirpation of a piece of the cerebral cortex can disappear amazingly fast. In order to explain this experience, numerous hypotheses have been established, all of which are absolutely unsatisfactory and to a large extent irreconcilable with clearly observable facts. If it is alleged that the destroyed cortex substance could regenerate, any anatomic proof for such a hypothesis is missing. On the contrary, I can demonstrate that, after the mutilation of the cerebrum, the rest of the brain shrinks. Therefore, there remains no choice but to conclude that the restoration of the lost function is taken over by a part of the brain that was not destroyed. But any such supposition clearly contradicts the basis of the entire localization doctrine. For, if a center that performs a special function should be able to take over the function of another, destroyed center with a different function, then the same section of the brain obviously executes different functions at the same time. Once the possibility of such an adjustment is admitted for the mutilated animal, it cannot be conceived not to exist also in the uninjured. If, for example, a dog who is blind as a result of the removal of the vision center governing both sides learns to see again later, one should not, however, be permitted to maintain that the tail-center or the taste-center should suddenly also govern the vision-center, and if one sets up such an assumption any-how, then one gives up the entire basic principle of the localization doctrine. In order to avoid this embarrassment, Munk has chosen a new amazing alternative. He supposes that each center with a specific function is, in a certain way, surrounded by a nonactive fallow-land of virginal cortex substance that only starts to function as a substi-tution when the center usually employed is destroyed by chance. Ac-cording to this strange theory, we would thus possess an extraordi-nary surplus of available brain substance in order to be protected against the possibility of our suffering a mutilation of the brain. As artificial as such a hypothesis may appear, it is not even sufficient, as will be shown later. Considered closely, Hitzig and his successors are found to be in much closer agreement with the theories of Flourens than they would like to admit.

Flourens asserts that the cerebrum can be mutilated without caus-ing any impairment of its functions. Hitzig and his successors also teach that shortly after the mutilation of the cerebral cortex, no func-tional disturbance can be observed. The entire difference between the doctrine of Flourens and that of the modern localizationist is simply a matter of the time required for restitution. According to Flourens, restitution is supposed to occur immediately after muti-lation, whereas his opponents claim a certain, even though short, time for restitution of function after mutilation of the cerebrum. When my investigation of the function of the cerebrum began, about six years ago, it seemed most important to me to clarify this point, on which Flourens agreed with the more recent experimental scientists. It seemed hardly believable to me that the larger part of the cerebrum should actually be totally superfluous, since suppos-edly with time a total restitution takes place following mutilation. In an extended sequence of tests I accomplished the task of causing most extensive destructions of the cerebral cortex and at the same time keeping the animals alive as long as possible for observation. In order to avoid bleeding, I flushed out the cerebral substance with a jet of water.

The main result of this sequence of tests was proof that Flourens's doctrine, according to which a small residue of the cerebrum is still capable of executing all the functions of the cerebrum, rests on an error. An extensive destruction of both hemispheres always causes conspicuous, permanent disturbances of the higher psychical activities of the animal, especially a reduction of intelligence. All of my predecessors, with the exception of Ferrier, had, strangely enough, not mentioned this phenomenon at all. Judging from the assertions made by Hitzig and his predecessors, one would have thought that the cerebrum brings about the movements of the limbs, the muscle-sense, seeing, hearing, etc., but that it has nothing to do with the functions on the basis of which we deduce intelligence. Before me, only Ferrier declared that the frontal lobes, part of the cerebrum, preside over what we call intelligence. But I have very carefully exempted the frontal lobes of my dogs in most cases and only destroyed the parietal and occipital lobes, and still I have observed, especially with these animals, the most prominent disturbance of their intelligence. Therefore, it cannot be maintained that the frontal lobes must be considered as the main center of intelligence.

In the cases of dogs with extensive flushing of the cerebrum I was able, in addition, during the period following each operation, regularly to observe the same motor disturbances as have been accurately described by old and new authors. If the flushing affects one hemisphere, the animals are paralyzed on one side for the first few days, hemiplegically. But soon the hemiplegia recedes and in a matter of weeks the dogs run around using all of their limbs, like healthy dogs. I could further confirm, in agreement with Hitzig and Ferrier, that, after an extensive one-sided destruction of the cerebral cortex, a dog is blind on the opposite-side eye for the first few days. But this blindness is only temporary. If it is possible to keep the animal alive, it will then learn to see again; but after extensive damage it will show a very peculiar disturbance in its visual perception. Such a dog will, with great certainty, avoid obstacles when walking. In this respect it thus makes a very practical use of its visual impressions. But the animal is no longer frightened when it is threatened with a fist or a whip. It is apathetic at the sight of people or strange animals. It does not recognize food thrown to him and can find it only very slowly. Munk, who later confirmed this disturbance of the visual perception that I discovered, has introduced the term "psychic blindness" for this phenomenon. But, since adopting this term might erroneously suggest that I accept the fantastic explanation Munk has given for this condition, I prefer to reject this term. Therefore I suggest calling the perceptional disturbance I discovered cerebral blindness, or, even better, cerebral feebleness of vision.

The permanent disturbances of the remaining sensory perceptions after extensive mutilation of both hemispheres are of a much less evident nature, so that they escaped me at the beginning, when my attention was captured by the very obvious manifestations of cerebral feebleness of vision. Later I proved that all sensory perceptions show permanent anomalies. The animals with extensive loss of substance in both hemispheres do still hear, for they make movements when a loud noise is produced in their vicinity, but they do not react to sound impressions in the same way they did before the operation. For example, they no longer bark when someone knocks at the door and no longer join in when other dogs bark. They also no longer know how to orient themselves with the aid of sound perceptions. When called, they often run off in a totally different direction. The faculty to perceive through scent or taste is also permanently damaged after an extensive mutilation of the cerebrum. Such dogs do not refuse to eat dogmeat, whereas a healthy dog disgustedly turns away from it. Tobacco smoke and chloroform vapor, for which normal dogs show the greatest disgust, are inhaled by the mutilated dogs with comparative equanimity. Finally, I have also found that the perceptions transmitted through the skin are duller in every respect for such dogs. They still have a perceptive faculty in all points of the skin, but they only react to strong stimuli. They do not mind remaining with their feet in cold water for a long time, express pain only after intense pressure on the skin, and do not find their way easily by groping.

Thus the permanent functional disturbances after extensive mutilation of the cerebrum—not known before my work, because nobody kept the animals alive as long—consist of an impairment of intelligence with strange impairments of all sensory perceptions. I have called these permanent impairments deficiency manifestations because they are caused by the loss of a large portion of the cerebral cortex. I attribute the highest importance to these deficiency manifestations. The temporary disorders that last only a short time after the operation and then disappear seem of lesser importance to me. I believe that these cannot be deduced from the removal of the cerebral cortex because then they could not be evened out so fast. I suppose rather that deeper nerve centers that are not directly damaged nevertheless experience a temporary restriction of their functions. When, with the healing of the wound, the restriction disappears, the centers paralyzed only temporarily take up their functions again, and the surprising establishment of apparently lost functions becomes evident.

This explanation, which rests primarily on analogous experiences occurring after injury of the spinal cord, has been attacked by many. But the recognition seems to break through more and more that it is advisable to distinguish between permanent and transient manifestations after injuries of the cerebrum.

The experiments just described were at first pursued only to obtain clarity on the question of restitution; but the results obtained justify immediate expression of the most serious doubts about all the modern localization doctrines by which the cerebral cortex is divided into small, delineated fields with separate functions. I had never tried to cause exact symmetrical lesions during my operations, but nevertheless the disturbances were always amazingly similar on both sides of the body. Whenever I observed very pronounced impairment in visual perception after mutilation of the cerebral cortex, all the remaining sensory perceptions were also damaged. This did not seem reconcilable with the hypothesis of strictly defined centers for each sense.

When these and other considerations forced me to conclude that the hypotheses of Hitzig, Ferrier, and their successors could not possibly be correct, this did not exclude, of course, the possibility that some totally different kind of spatial distribution of cerebral functions does actually exist. In fact, I have been accused of denying any localization of cerebral function, but that is wrong. I absolutely believe it possible that the individual cortices of such a powerful organ as the cerebrum have varying functions. But whether and to what extent this possibility proves true, that will remain to be investigated, dispassionately investigated. . . . [Omitted are paragraphs that deal with the details of his experiments and the conclusions he has come to.]

Having brought my work on the question of restitution to a sufficient completion, I have tried in the course of the last two years to actively address the localization problem, which I had only touched on critically and occasionally. Since the flushing out method seemed inappropriate to me to cause clearly delineated losses of substance, I chose another method. I used the drill invented by White, with which I put small instruments I devised into fast rotations. . . . In each operation I have removed at most the fourth of the cerebral cortex observable from above. In the case of some dogs, I have conducted two, three, four, and more operations and have carefully observed the resulting manifestations of deficiencies.

A dog that has lost both frontal quadrants—that is, the excitable zones of both sides—will be permanently idiotic. The observer immediately notices a stupid expression in the eyes. Such a dog, who according to Ferrier should have lost the so-called psychomotor centers, according to Munk the sensory sphere, and according to Hitzig muscle consciousness, runs around in lively fashion, moves the lower jaws, the tongue, the tail, eyes, ears, thus shows no paralysis at all, although immediately after the operation he had a distinct weakness in the opposite side's limbs. At all points of his body the dog has sensory perceptions, although they are dull. He also has muscle consciousness in the sense Hitzig conceived this term; for he will not let his paws be put in just any position without soon moving them back. With Munk one could perhaps object by saying that at first the disturbances actually occurring after the removal of the so-called motor centers fade because these centers, or sensory spheres, as he calls them, have not been destroyed deeply enough. To confront this alibi, I have . . . made deep incisions, being able to keep even these animals alive. Although the hemiplegia was of rather long duration in these cases, it disappeared almost completely and a few weeks later these animals could not be distinguished from those that had suffered lesions only five millimeters deep—not lesions of several centimeters! I therefore have to affirm that my experiences cannot be reconciled with the doctrines of Hitzig, Ferrier, and Munk. The only permanent motor disturbance I observed in dogs from which both the parietal lobes had been removed was that they move more clumsily and cannot keep a bone in their front paws while nibbling on it.

A dog whose posterior quadrants—that is, what Hitzig calls the nonexcitable zone—are destroyed on both sides, as far as visible from above, always appears much more idiotic than ones whose parietal lobes have been removed. This is probably adequately explained by the fact that the entire cortex of the posterior lobe has a much larger circumference than the cortex of the parietal lobe. According to Hitzig and Munk, such a dog should be totally blind, because he has lost his whole visual sphere. But this is absolutely not the case. Such animals show signs of cerebral feebleness of vision—for example, they do not respond to threatening gestures—but they can avoid obstacles and even recognize an approaching human from a certain distance. Besides the cerebral feebleness of vision they also suffer impaired perceptions based on scent, taste, or hearing. These experiences prove that Munk's so-called visual sphere does not exclusively serve the visual sense in the first place and, in the second place, that animals can have visual perception without a visual sphere.

Signs of impairment can be amazingly insignificant for a dog from which only one side of the gray cortex has been largely removed. The animal whose skull I am showing you here, and whose cerebrum is represented in a drawing I will present to you, had a scarcely impaired intelligence. Although he seemed to prefer to use his left eye, when this was closed by us, we realized that he was still able to see very well, showed fear when threatened, perceived meat from afar, etc.

Although even the substantial destruction of the cortex of one hemisphere scarcely damaged the intelligence, the intelligence is reduced to an extraordinary degree when the loss involves both hemispheres and is, moreover, large. The dog whose skull I am showing you here had survived four major operations and was only killed a year after the last operation. This dog was markedly idiotic and acted only like a reflexive eating machine. He paid no attention to humans or animals. All his sensory perceptions were severely damaged, but we observed that all his senses still functioned. He was neither deaf nor blind nor deprived of his gustatory or olfactory senses. Not a muscle of his body was paralyzed, not a point of his skin deprived of sensory perception. The cerebrum of this animal, hardened in Müller's fluid, weighs only 13 grams, whereas the cerebrum of a healthy animal, hardened in the same fluid, weighs 90 grams. As a result of the removal of the cortex, a very obvious secondary shrinking of the remaining cerebrum had taken place.

[Goltz then described the dog he brought from Strasbourg that had undergone five operations between November 15, 1880, and May 25, 1881, in the course of which the cortices of both parietal and occipital lobes had been removed. The frontal and temporal lobes were not touched. The dog represented one of his most interesting cases because of his lively movements, since generally dogs with extensive cerebral defects were very apathetic. Goltz described the behavior of the dog when his box was opened and when he moved around. Very often he raised himself, without support of his front paws, onto his hind legs and walked around. The dog manifested peculiar disturbances of sensory perceptions: it had an idiotic expression in its eyes, no reaction to a finger held in front of his eyes, and no expression of fear when threatened by a whip, a fist, an angry cat, or a burning candle. Although the dog was not blind, as proved by the fact that he could tell when the cover of his box was removed and that he avoided obstacles put in his way and sometimes even avoided imagined obstacles. But he had been deprived, for example, of his instinct to choose a warm spot to rest on. The dog thus showed explicitly the perceptual deficiencies that Goltz had described as cerebral feebleness of vision. Later, in the afternoon session of the congress, Goltz introduced the dog itself.]

Our dog hears, but he responds to sound impressions very differently than other dogs. He does not express fear when yelled at or when a whip is cracked. He never joins in when other dogs bark. The dog now eats dogmeat without any disgust. He also shows no dislike of tobacco smoke or chloroform vapor. He has sensory perceptions on all points of his skin. It was not necessary to investigate this fact any further because we had a little, lively dog, quite young, which loved to play. As soon as it was left with the feeble-minded dog, the latter let himself be attacked in a playful way and even played with the little dog on occasions. But when the little dog bit him more seriously, he made loud noises of pain, got angry, and tried to bite the little dog. Once he was angry, he would repel any further attacks of the small dog, growling and baring his teeth. By means of these observations, we made sure that mechanical abuse of the skin at any point of this animal causes expressions of pain and actions of defense.

Our dog is much less idiotic than was the animal whose cerebrum weighed only 13 grams. He is friendly to humans, cares little about other dogs except for traces of sexual drive, shows his contentment when let out, his discontent when locked up, shows no envy, and lets other dogs take things away from him. He has retained the instinct of hiding his food and then later eating the hidden food when he is hungry again.

These descriptions are sufficient to prove that the animal has to be considered a harmlessly idiotic being. Another experiment we conducted explains how much this dog has lost what we call intelligence. Placed in a spot surrounded by a very low fence, he cannot figure out how to climb over it, although the fence only reaches up to his breast. In his box he pulls himself up along a barrier that is much higher than the fence. But he does not find the means to overcome the obstacle as he does in his box. He is too dumb to do that.

The autopsy of the cerebrum will show to what extent the cortex of this animal has been destroyed. It is possible that somewhere a border portion of the so-called visual sphere on one or both sides has been spared. With forced efforts the proponents of the localization doctrine would then want to ascribe the visual functions this animal still possesses to the retained sparse remains of the visual sphere. But it will be more difficult, if one wishes to insist on the localization hypotheses, to demonstrate why this animal also reacts differently than a normal dog to impressions of hearing and scent, when his auditory and olfactory spheres have not been attacked directly.

It seems totally impossible to me to make the actual observations obtained with this dog agree with all those localization hypotheses that have been established in connection with the so-called excitable zone; if Munk's doctrine, which posits that his so-called sensory sphere is in the excitable zone, had only a shadow of a foundation, then the dog would have to be numb on large portions of the skin of both halves of the body. He would have had to retain sensation only on the regions of the skin the sensory spheres of which were not destroyed. But we were able to convince ourselves that the animal has a sense of touch not only at the skin of the trunk, whose sensory sphere it still possesses, but also at the head, the limbs, and the tail; for it defends itself by biting against injury of these parts of the body.

It is equally easy to prove that this dog has muscle-consciousness in the sense of Hitzig even though he has lost the centers of the muscle-consciousness. In no way is he indifferent against the position of his paws but returns them to the original comfortable position immediately when they have been placed artificially into a divergent position.

Finally, with respect to the proponents of the psychomotor centers, it has to be pointed out that this dog, even though he has been deprived in both hemispheres of at least a large number of those centers, is nevertheless able to move all his muscles apparently voluntarily.

He does not only execute the general, more machine-like motions of walking and running but, as we can see, he is also capable of raising himself on his hind legs. He bites when he plays with a dog. He shows his content by wagging his tail. He often methodically scratches his head and other parts of the body. In addition, he tries to get rid of a cap that is put over his head in order to close his eyes, by stripping it off with both front paws. One would not want to call these actions simple reflex movements, however.

As I have described, our dog really has some motor disturbances. His movements are clumsier than the ones of healthy dogs. He slips easily and acts awkwardly in certain operations: He does not know how to hold fast to a bone with his paws. These disturbances seem to be the only ones that regularly remain after extensive mutilation of the sliding lobes (*Schleifenlappen*).

Thus the experiments we did with this animal have confirmed the hypotheses I established earlier:

1. The cortex of the cerebrum is the organ of the higher psychic activities. Upon removal of large parts of both halves of the cerebrum, the intelligence is reduced.

2. It is impossible to paralyze any muscle by destroying any one portion of the cerebral cortex. The mutilated animal retains the voluntary use of all muscles.

3. It is equally impossible to destroy any sensory activity permanently by destroying any one portion of the cerebral cortex. The animal retains all his senses. But after the removal of extensive portions of the cerebral cortex, weakness of perception occurs.

4. Animals with destroyed parietal lobes have clumsier movements permanently and duller cutaneous perception than the animals with destroyed occipital lobes. Dogs with destroyed occipital lobes are in general more idiotic than animals that have only lost their parietal lobes.

Afternoon Session

[After some discussion of Goltz's theories, the members of the section travel that afternoon to King's College to observe Goltz and Ferrier demonstrate their experimental animals.]

Gentlemen! I herewith introduce the dog who has made the trip from Strasbourg to London with me. The animal has lost by far the largest portion of the cortex substance of both parietal lobes and both occipital lobes, as I described it to you this morning. Of the five operations that resulted in this enormous mutilation of the cerebrum, the last one took place on May 25 of this year. The deformation of the skull of the animal is very obvious. If I hold his head, you can easily put several fingers next to each other into each of the enormous cavities on both sides.

Upon letting the dog roam around freely, you will see him wag his tail in a lively manner, walking to and fro, avoiding obstacles carefully. The movements of the four limbs are generally absolutely normal. Sometimes the animal slides, and that happens more often involving the hind paws than the front paws. Once in a while the dog hits objects with the left side of his body. In the movement of his limbs, of the head, the ears, the tongue, and the tail no trace of asymmetry can be observed.

We now want to examine the individual sensory functions and observe to what extent they show anomalies.

The position of the eyes of the dog shows no deviation. The pupils contract well upon the stimulation by light. When the animal moves his eyes, the muscles of both eyeballs act together as they should. But you will notice that the expression of the eyes is fixed, stupid. An intelligent dog concentrates his gaze at the eyes of the person looking at him. Our dog does not do that.

The fact that the dog can see is proven by his avoidance of obstacles. But visual impressions do not at all produce the same manifestations as in the case of unmutilated dogs. I threaten him now with my fist, while he approaches me wagging his tail in a friendly manner. You see that he does not pay any attention to the threat, but instead continues to wag his tail. I now take up this whip and move it back and forth, as if I wanted to beat the animal with it. But the dog does not show any signs of fear in face of the threatening whip. Just as little does he notice a burning candle. Whereas a healthy dog runs off or at least turns his head away, our dog remains completely impassive and does not even twinkle his eyelids if we bring the flame of the candle close to his eyes. You can see, therefore, that this animal is not moved to any motor reactions from which we could conclude that he has any reactions of fear, fright, interest, or curiosity. This dog remains indifferent and apathetic in the face of visual impressions. In my discussion of this morning I told you that this dog even avoids imagined obstacles. I observed that, when walking around, he avoided a spot lit brightly by the sun. Because of this experience I made the following experiment with him. I had a flag sewn that consists of a glaringly white, broad strip of linen bordered by two black strips. If we put this flag on the ground, the dog avoids stepping on the white strip. I have brought the flag along and shall dare to repeat the test here.

(The lecturer spreads the flag on the floor of the hall. The strolling dog walks around the flag for several minutes. As soon as the flag has been removed, the animal soon steps again on the part of the floor that it avoided before.)

That the actions of this dog are governed by his visual impressions is, in addition, proved convincingly by the fact that his whole behavior changes when his eyes are artificially closed. I brought a cap along that I will put over his head. Thus no beam of light can now reach his eyes. You see how the animal, which earlier avoided all obstacles, now hits his head repeatedly. You observe how he tries to pull off the cap with both his front paws. We are now taking off the cap and we see that he takes up his wanderings in the same way as before the cap was put on his head.

Our dog is just as little deaf as blind. But he does react to sound impressions in a different way than an uninjured animal. See how he stands right in front of me. I scream at him: "Be off! Move! Get away!" He does not flee, he does not give evidence of fear by any movement. Just as little can he be intimidated by the crack of a whip. (The lecturer strongly cracks a whip.) You see that the animal continues to wag his tail in a friendly manner. But you could perceive that the dog did hear the intense sound itself when he, immediately after the crack of the whip, made a movement with his head that could be interpreted as something like a sign of amazement. I will try to call him over to me. You see that he heard my call, for he was at first startled and now keeps a faster pace, but the animal does not know how to choose the proper direction towards me, and errs around aimlessly.

This animal still possesses the faculty of smelling. When meeting other animals, it still shows a sexual drive. He knows how to find pieces of meat thrown to him by smelling them out. But you can see for yourself that he does not react to olfactory impressions as distinctly as an uninjured dog. He licks the human hand extended to him, but licks the face of a living cat held before him in a similar way.

Cigarette smoke, which is disagreeable to healthy dogs, leaves him quite unconcerned. (One of the gentlemen present lights a cigar and blows the smoke against the nose of the dog. The dog does not flee and turns his head only when very thick smoke is blown at him.)

The cutaneous perception of the animal seems to be somewhat dulled all over, but it cannot be doubted at all that this dog possesses sensory perception at all points of the outer skin and the mucous membranes. He reacts to very intense injury of the surface skin with signs of displeasure. It seems almost superfluous to support this fact by an experiment, but I will perform one anyhow in order to show you this little instrument that Mr. Ewald has constructed. This aesthesiometer permits exposure of a part of the body, for example a paw, to increasing pressure. The instrument also contains a device that makes it possible to immediately release the pressure. When using this instrument, the pressure is increased up to the point when the animal shows a definite sensory manifestation, and then the squeezing tool is immediately released by a manual manipulation. We are now putting the left hind paw into the apparatus. With a slight tightening of the screw that causes the increase of the pressure, the animal squeals and tries to get loose.

From what I have told you, you will have, as I have, won the conviction that this dog has to be judged as being harmlessly idiotic. He still possesses all his senses, but he does not know how to utilize his sensory perceptions as efficiently as an uninjured animal. Therefore, he is also not capable of providing any samples of reflection. He cannot cope with the smallest embarrassment. I will show you this by means of a very simple experiment. We have put up here a small enclosed fence, the height of which is so minimal that it reaches only to the breast of the animal. We are now putting the dog into the enclosure and will try to entice him by a call to climb over the fence. You see that the animal paces up and down within the enclosure, knocks against everything with his breast, bends his head over the fence, but can absolutely not reach the decision to climb over the very low fence. You may now believe that the animal is altogether not able to get up on his hind legs. But that is absolutely erroneous, as I will prove immediately. I now put the dog into this deep case in which he has spent the trip to London. As soon as I will have removed the cover without any noise, the dog will immediately appear, raising himself on his hind legs, and will put his front paws on the rim of the case wall. (The lecturer opens the case, and the dog shows himself immediately.) The wall of this case is more than twice as high as the enclosure. [I believe that I] have shown that this dog does not show any kind of paralysis. His movements are somewhat clumsy and awkward, but he executes the most varying movements. Thus the dog would easily get out of the enclosure if he would employ the same muscle effort within the enclosure as was familiar to him in the case. No muscle is deprived of voluntary use. Thus he has to be classified as idiotic because he does not know how to use such a simple resource at his disposition in order to free himself from his dilemma.

Thus closing my demonstrations, gentlemen, I hope that, in addition, you have satisfied yourself about the fact that no sensory function of this animal has ceased to exist. It can see, hear, smell, feel. But the dog shows most noteworthy deviations in his attitude toward sensory perceptions. His actions are so inept, yes, partly even absurd, that there is no denying that he is devoid of the faculty of reflection and has to be declared idiotic.

The dog will be killed by chloroform within the next few days and then you will be able to see for yourself, by personal observation, the immense extent of the injury.

Appendix B: Panizza

A problem remains still for the physiologist that, however, is relevant mostly to pathology. The effects of a stimulus tend to become generalized in the organism, and this conforms both to the teachings of anatomy on the connections of all the parts of this system and to the nature of excitability common to all those parts. But this does not always happen; rather, such effects are limited more often to single areas. If we then consider a certain number of cases in which a certain point on the nervous system has been injured, above all in the centers we can observe a relationship between the injuries and the peripheral parts that are affected by them, which by reason of its constancy has allowed the birth of an illusion of absolute constancy. Thus, for example, an injury in a cerebral hemisphere limits its effects to only one side of the body, which can be the same or opposite side on which the injury occurred. However, the statistics show that a greater number of cases of paralysis took place following an injury to one hemisphere, both to the other side and to the same side as the injury. Thus a direct connection by means of independent nerve fibers can no longer be argued, nor [a connection] between the injured part and the area showing the paralysis. We can no longer explain the crossing effect by means of a decussation, nor can we explain the numerous exceptions by means of anomalous anatomical structures in which the effect is missing. Therefore we must search elsewhere for the reasons for these facts.

What we deduce from the facts is contrary to the theory of localization.

Given these considerations, it is clear that the fact of partial sensory and motor paralysis following an injury to the nerve centers can never be brought up as proof that either sensitivity or the instigating principle of movement is located in the injured spot. In order to be used as proof, it would be necessary for no other area to be injured and give rise to the same effects, and for the same effects always to follow the injury of the same area with absolute constancy. But such constancy is universally contradicted by the facts. Not only can the irritation of *any* point on the nervous system give rise to the same morbid phenomena identical to those obtained by irritating areas that are far apart and totally different, but the most varied phenomena can be obtained by irritating the same point: "Very numerous experiences," writes Brown-Séquard, "which confirm the teachings of human pathology have proved to me that producing the same injury in the same area of animals of the same species can give rise, as in man, to an immense variety of effects."[1]

Suggested hypotheses to Reconcile the Facts with the Theory of Localization

Thus the physiologists who would like to assign a place in the cerebral centers to sensitivity and to will cannot derive any experimental proof from these facts. But in truth it cannot be said that any of them have ever made this claim; their efforts have been turned only toward the search for hypotheses that would reconcile the mass of facts, which they themselves recognize as contrary to the localization theory, with the theory itself.

Indirect paralyses. All cases in which an irritation of peripheral areas has given rise to paralytic phenomena in distant organs has been explained by saying that it was a case of indirect paralysis, that is to say, it was supposed that the condition of irritation was not only diffused through the nerves or through peripheral ganglial centers, but that it first ran to the centers where the sensitivity and motility of the paralyzed organ is localized, and that its influence was shown on them. Thus, for example, in the case in which a wound to the sciatic nerve produces a paralysis of the upper limb on the same side, the cause of paralysis would have gone directly to the cerebral centers to interrupt the action of those nerves which determine the movement of that limb. Even if we suppose independent centripetal routes of conduction, the connection of various cerebral centers and the different degree of resistance that they can oppose to the diffusion of the stimulus would explain up to a certain point the variety of these effects. We must, however, point out that we are dealing with a hypothesis adjusted to support a theory, but one that does not prove at all the existence of the centers.

Flourens's hypothesis. It has been more difficult to reconcile with the theory, the facts that demonstrate that the extended injuries of the cerebral hemispheres present neither sensitivity nor movement. And it is on these facts that the skill of the physiologists has for the most part applied itself. Flourens had said that the cerebral hemispheres were the only sensing parts of the organism, meaning by this that they were the parts to which impressions had to arrive in order for the animal to be aware of them. The animal deprived of its hemispheres was thus deprived of all sensitivity and was compared by Flourens to a man deeply alseep.[2] Cuvier, however, pointed out that a man immersed in sleep, who moves, who assumes a more comfortable position, cannot be said not to have sensations, but rather should be described as "one who has neither the distinct impression nor the memory of it."[3] Flourens accepted the distinction and later wrote, "The animal that has lost its cerebral lobes has not lost its sensitivity; it still has it completely; it has lost only the perception of sensation; it has lost only its intelligence.[4] It is therefore psychology that comes to the aid of physiology. Psychology made intelligence out to be a faculty that elaborates the material furnished by sensations, and one that is totally distinct and independent from the sense of touch; the physiologist assigned separate areas in the brain to the two faculties. Cuvier said, "The cerebral lobes are the receptacle in which all sensations take distinct shape and leave lasting imprints; they are the seat of memory, the faculty with which they provide the animal with material for judgment."[5] Longet says that "the physiologist must be allowed to distinguish simple perception, which is in a certain way crude, of impressions, from the attention paid to them, and from the tendency to form ideas in relation with them."[6] Vulpian says similarly, "Such perception, as it must be understood in physiology (that is, Longet's "simple or crude perception," sensation) certainly takes place outside of the brain; but it is in the brain that the work of isolating different sensations from each other, of appreciating them at their proper value, of analyzing them, of transforming them into ideas, takes place."[7] Lussana and Lemoigne say, "With sensation, the animal perceives the physical qualities of objects (contact, resistance, odors, flavors, light, sounds); with perception, the animal transforms these different sensations into ideas relative to intelligence and instinctual impulses (food, drink, danger, companionship, enemy, space, place, time, etc.)."[8] We shall not now criticize the concept of faculty understood thus, which already presents itself as an empty abstraction, but we shall consider the hypothesis only from the perspective of physiology.

This distinction and this differing localization of the two faculties having been established, the physiologist used to explain how sensitivity and movements are not destroyed after the demolition of the cerebral hemispheres: only the intelligence, which has its seat in the hemispheres, is destroyed, and thus only the movements that respond to the ideas are destroyed; but the movements that respond to sensations still remain, since sensitivity is outside the hemispheres. [William B.] Carpenter explains it thus: "The movements that are observed in animals with an intact nervous system are ideomotor and sensorimotor reactions; in animals that are deprived of their brains, they are simply sensorimotor reactions." It must be pointed out that there is no fact that serves to effectively differentiate these two types of movement: after removal of the brain, the animals perform movements identical to those they performed when the nervous system was whole. It is only the interpretation of this fact that varies according

to the ideas professed by single authors. If a frog deprived of its cerebral hemispheres is thrown into a pond, it can be seen to begin
swimming with totally normal movements, to reach shore, to leave
the water, and to assume the position of rest. It could be supposed
that the frog is still capable of voluntary movements: "A particular
excitation," says Vulpian on the other hand, "of the entire surface of
the body is produced upon contact with the water; this excitation ini-
tiates the swimming mechanism, and this mechanism ceases to act as
soon as the cause of excitation is also removed when the animal has
left the water."[9] But it is easy to see that the stimulus here has initiated
not only the swimming mechanism, but also the mechanism of the
animals' efforts to climb out on the bank to leave the water. Vulpian
could not avoid making this observation: "I can see very well," he
adds, "something singular in the series of movements by which the
frog leaves the water and climbs up on the banks of the pond to resume its position of rest; but instead of seeing here a proof of the
persistence of the animals' will, I see here a proof of the extent of the
power of the excitomotor stimulations in animals."[10] In other words,
the physiologist sees in these facts, which always stay the same, what
is convenient to him or what he chooses to see.

To support the hypothesis, the differences that can reflect the actions of two animals of the same species, in which one has undergone
the removal of the brain and the other is left intact, have been greatly
exaggerated. The state of somnolence or stupor or amnesia in which
the former falls compared with the latter has been overstressed. It has
also been noted that the movements of the former are less lively. Vulpian writes, "These movements lack that quality of random spontaneity that can be observed in intact animals, which cause them to
be considered voluntary movements."[11] But it can have occurred to
nobody who has doubts about localization, as far as I know, to declare
a perfect identity between an intact animal and an animal of the same
species that has been deprived of its brain. The sole effects of such a
grave trauma would suffice to place the two animals in conditions
much different from each other. But such vague differences are not a
valid argument for the localization exclusively in the brain of intelligence and will, and it is certain that we do not have experimental data
that can demonstrate that an animal deprived of its brain is deprived
of consciousness. Goltz puts two frogs in a vessel full of water, one

frog being decapitated and the other only blinded to impede the production of voluntary movements that would follow visual impressions. At the time of immersion the water is at 25° C. It is slowly
warmed to 50° C. Now Goltz says that he has observed that the second
frog attempts to escape and shows signs of distress from the beginning and dies when the temperature reaches 42°, and that the other
remains calmer and gives no signs of distress or pain, and dies when
the temperature reaches 50°. The calmness of the decapitated frog was
not, however, absolute; Goltz himself admits that it made defensive
movements analogous to those of the frog to whose skin acetic acid
was applied. We have repeated this experiment numerous times and
have reached totally opposite results, which, in order not to negate
Goltz's statements, forces us to think that he made the experiment
only one time, and that in this time, as an exception, the shock of
decapitation had immobilized the animal, or had greatly handicapped
its sensorimotor reactions. When two frogs, under the same conditions, have been placed in a vessel of water at 25° C, we have *always*
observed that the blinded frog floated there calmly with its head out
of the water until the heat went over 35°. At the same time the decapitated frog was agitated, swimming in every direction, and made repeated attempts to jump out of the water; in one instance, the frog
jumped out of the vessel twice. When the temperature had reached
42°, the decapitated frog always died, as did the blinded frog a few
minutes later, and both in the same manner, with general trembling
and convulsive movements.[12]

When we see that Ferrier finds in Goltz's experiment the proof
"*most conclusive* that a frog without a brain and capable of reflex acts
is perfectly insensible to stimulations that in a normal state give rise
to symptoms of pain,"[13] we can thus verify the strength of a precon-
ceived idea even in the face of the clearest evidence. The same hypothesis proves insufficient in light of other facts. The hypothesis
does not explain the cases recorded from human pathology in which
the complete or partial destruction of a hemisphere did not destroy
or disturb any of these manifestations that are considered necessarily
tied to intelligence. Thus, for example, Smoler observed in the Clinic
of Halla the complete suppuration of a hemisphere in an individual
who had taken a long walk and had carried several buckets of water
to a fourth floor a few hours before dying.[14]

Further, this hypothesis does not explain the results of those experiments that demonstrate that an animal becomes paralyzed immediately after the destruction of one hemisphere, but resumes shortly afterwards the use of all its faculties. Many animals, one of whose cerebral hemispheres has been removed, do not differ, as were observed by all experimenters, from intact animals. In some, however, disturbances of locomotion were observed, and also, particularly in dogs, paralysis of the front legs; but these disturbances were temporary and, with the healing of the wound, the animals were observed to resume their former state. If, when the brain was entirely removed, one could attribute the significance of sensorimotor reactions to actions performed, there is no sign here that the removal of one hemisphere disturbs or suppresses intelligence. Gall had already supposed that the same faculty resided in symmetrical points of both hemispheres, and that therefore the surviving hemisphere could substitute for the other destroyed hemisphere by itself. But we can remove from an animal corresponding parts of the two hemispheres, proceeding from front to back or from back to front, or from top to bottom, and after the operation the animal will not differ in any way from an intact animal.

These experiments were performed first by Flourens, then by Longet, by Vulpian, and by many other experimenters, always with the same results. Vulpian removed the anterior part of the cerebral lobes from a frog and observed that, during the scarring, the frog hunted a fly placed in front of it but could not reach it with its tongue in one shot; after some time had passed, the frog would capture it at the first try, and at the end the frog differed from an intact frog only in being less lively and in being less eager to escape.[15] But there are also pathological facts in man that could be cited as evidence against Gall's hypothesis. Trousseau saw a man who had been wounded by a bullet entering one temple and exiting through the other, and who, for three months (that is, until he died), kept not only his intelligence intact, but preserved as well his peaceful and lively disposition.[16] Velpeau tells of an individual whose two cerebral hemispheres were destroyed in their anterior part to the extent of about four centimeters and had been replaced by a hard, fibrous, bilobal tumor, each lobe of which was as big as a hen's egg, which originated from the *dura mater*; the surrounding cerebral matter was furthermore red and soft. Before dying, this individual was in a totally normal condition and, in fact, was quite talkative.[17]

Vulpian also mentions a man, the anterior portions of whose cranium had been penetrated by a bullet, with the escape of a large quantity of cerebral matter, who for four months was shown to be in possession of his intelligence, speaking without any difficulty.[18] Other similar cases are mentioned by Longet.[19] Flourens, faced with facts of this kind, thought that intellectual processes were possible even with a very limited portion of the hemispheres, and that intelligence would be abolished only with their complete and total destruction. This faculty, according to Flourens, was made possible, on the one hand, by means of the hemispheres, but on the other hand was essentially single, so that with one portion of the hemispheres destroyed, this faculty would retreat into the surviving portion, and if destruction were continued, would retreat further into the remaining cerebral matter until no trace of it would be left. Only then would it disappear.[20] Vulpian does not find another resource to reconcile the facts with localization of intelligence in the hemispheres, except for this hypothesis: "Cerebral functions," he concludes, "can still be carried out even with a very limited portion of the hemispheres."[21] Carville and Duret also accept this hypothesis, which was called "substitution" or "functional replacement." It is evident that physiological criticism would never have been able to reach a doctrine within these premises, but if other physiologists did not accept this, it is because they had different psychological bases.

Ferrier's hypothesis. According to a more recent psychology, it seemed that the faculties, as understood by the authors quoted above, were not, in the final analysis, anything but sensations. Certain physiologists accepted this view more gladly, not so much because sensation, as a subjective element deriving from the modification of a nerve cell, is something arising from experience, but because it turned out to be easier to understand the relationships of the nervous system with the psychological element, relationships that were inconceivable with the abstractions of older psychology.

In other words, the problem could not be solved by reducing the entire psychological sphere to pure sensation—that is, What does a sensation consist of?—but it was thought that this perspective at least allowed the establishment of the nature of the psychological condition that invariably accompanies a predetermined exterior excitation. And this represented an improved point of view, since it concerned an area of research whose goal is to establish how elements are united; elements that, as Lotze declares, must be supposed to be self-contained and separate.[22] In the following chapters we will see how this psychological doctrine as well cannot be absolutely accepted by science. For now we must consider only to what conclusions this doctrine has brought the physiology of the nervous system.

Ferrier starts from these premises and considers sensations as the subjective side of the modification imprinted in the nerve cells by a present object.[23] But since this modification cannot be reproduced without the object being present, he then allows a reexcitability of the nerve cell, because of which sensation already received can be presented again to consciousness. "Sensation," says Ferrier, "becomes thus idealized," and he adds: "Perception, and thus the *idea* of an object, is the renewal of cellular modifications in each of the centers that have contributed to the process of knowing."[24] A sensation's possibility of being renewed is what generates, according to the same author, judgments of analogy, agreement, difference: "The foundation," he says, "of the consciousness of agreement is the reexciting, with a present impression, of the same molecular operations that coincide with a past impression; the judgment of difference consists in the passage from one physical modification into another."[25] Feelings of pain and of pleasure that accompany sensations can be considered "the subjective impression of harmony or of physical discord between the organism and the influences that act upon it."[26] Therefore, in addition, "the sources of conscious activity, or the incitements of will, are present sensations or are revived by the idea, together with what accompanies them."[27]

It is now understood how the physiologist who starts from these premises cannot call sensation and perception two distinct faculties, nor assign separate organs in the nervous system to each one of them; he will necessarily find only sensory organs. Because it is always the same sensation that becomes idea and impulse, these various operations would be able to have no function other than that of sensation: "Since ideal or revived sensation," says Ferrier, "occupies the same areas as those activated during actual sensations, the revived feelings or emotions are localized in the same area."[28] And he concludes, "A sensory, ideational, and emotional center is one and the same thing."[29] Voluntary movements require the functional activity of certain centers that should determine the movements themselves, when artificially stimulated; these are the centers that, according to the theory, must be called motor centers.[30] Hence we must search in the brain only for sensory and motor centers. Ferrier does not explain why the brain must be the seat of these centers; he says only, "We can proceed from this fact, as if from a definitely acquired plan."[31] However, he goes even further with localization and places these centers exclusively in the cerebral cortex: "So that the impressions made on individual sensory organs may excite the subjective modification called sensation, they must reach the cells of their respective cortical centers and cause specific molecular changes there."[32]

The reason for this further localization is easier to guess. It is not because of the idea, already well known to science and later popularized by Gall, that a relationship exists between the surface area of an animal's hemispheres and its intelligence. This idea was abandoned after Leuret, Baillarger, and Dareste demonstrated that this relationship does not exist at all and that there are animals superior to other, much more intelligent animals (including man himself) as regards the number and size of the convolutions. The reason, rather, resides in the following: from the moment in which Hitzig and Fritsch discovered the excitability of the cerebral cortex, and the movements stimulated by electricity were interpreted as sensorimotor reactions, the centers of all movements and all sensations of which the organism is capable were found in a limited area of that cortex. Fritsch and Hitzig found in a very limited area of the parietal lobes of dogs the motor centers of the muscles of the face, neck, back, abdomen, tail, and limbs.[33]

Ferrier found in a much larger area, but one still limited to the lateral areas of the hemispheres (posteroparietal lobe and ascending circumvolution), the motor centers of the muscles of the face, tongue, mouth, biceps (which, according to the author, would have their own center in the ascending frontal circumvolution), and of all other muscles of upper and lower limbs.[34] Similarly, in a restricted area were found the centers corresponding to all possible modalities of sensation. Ferrier found in the fold the center of vision; in an upper point of the temporosphenoidal circumvolution he found the hearing center; in the lower part of the same lobe (*subiculum cornis ammonis* and related parts) he found the smell and taste centers. He assigns to the occipital lobes the centers of visceral sensations, but through simple conjecture. It is known that sexual appetite is stimulated by tactile sensations and, especially in certain animals, by particular odors. Ferrier thinks that "a region closely joined to the centers of tactile and olfactory sensations could be considered as a likely seat of the sensations that constitute sexual appetite."[35] Thus given, we see that not only do all the centers reside in the hemispheres, but also that a large part of them remains without purpose, as for example, the frontal lobes, the function of which no one has as yet managed to find. The sensory and motor centers were thus localized exclusively in the cerebral cortex, because they were all found here, and nothing remained to be localized in the other parts of the brain. Hence no other function was assigned to these parts but the one that remained available—that is, the function of "connecting the centers of the cortex with the periphery."[36]

As is easily foreseen, this way of understanding localizations had to meet difficulties even greater than those found by the preceding doctrines, in order to be reconciled with the facts. Here the destruction of a hemisphere should of necessity produce a permanent hemiplegia and abolish the intelligence, since it requires the participation of at least one hemisphere. Several cases of permanent hemiplegia, following a hemispheral lesion in man and in monkeys, are given to support the theory. There are others, however, such as those of Smoler mentioned here, which refute it absolutely; these are not now taken into consideration. But even in the cases of hemiplegia because of lesion in one hemisphere it is known that often intelligence is not in the least disturbed. Ferrier is therefore forced to return to Gall's hypothesis, that is, that one hemisphere can substitute for the other in these functions: "If one hemisphere is removed or destroyed through disease," he writes, "movement and sensation are abolished on one side; but mental operations can still be performed by the remaining hemisphere."[37] This hypothesis is contradicted, as we know, by all those facts that demonstrate that intelligence still exists even when corresponding parts of the two hemispheres are removed.[38] The total removal of the brain, according to the authors who profess this doctrine, completely abolishes sensitivity and voluntary movement in the two sides of the body, together with intelligence. They must therefore admit that all movements by animals deprived of the brain, those movements that had obliged other physiologists to assume sensory centers outside the brain, are because of a mere mechanism. Hence they deny, against all experience, the spontaneity of these movements, and they explain their coordination to jumping, swimming, running, crying, and defense by affirming that the mechanism itself is preset by nature to respond to predetermined stimulations by jumping, swimming, crying [etc.], and, what is more interesting, by removing those influences from oneself once the brain has been removed, they are no longer perceived as sensation but, in a state of consciousness, had to be perceived by the animal as bothersome or painful.

It is supposed that centers of even more complex automatic and special actions exist in the *medulla oblongata* and in the *mesencephalon*, and among these the reflected impression of emotion is included. Thus, according to Ferrier, "the jumping from side to side performed to avoid an obstacle of a frog deprived of a brain would only be the result of two simultaneous impressions, one on the leg, the other on the retina," and "the cry that a rabbit makes in the same circumstances, when its paw is pinched, would be a purely reflected phenomenon, which does not depend on any real sensation of pain."[39] But the question then arose: how could those actions, which in the wholeness of the nervous system require the intervention of consciousness in order to be performed, still be performed when consciousness is lacking because of the removal of the hemispheres? Ferrier answers with another hypothesis: he declares that this is possible only because *those actions are automatically organized in the basal ganglia.*

It has been seen how, according to Ferrier, the optic thalami and the striated bodies contain fibers that serve merely to connect the centers of the cortex with the periphery; however, they also contain gangliar matter. He then imagines that precisely this matter fulfills such an inexplicable function. An act that requires, in order to be performed, the awareness of the sensory impressions, becomes, because of frequent repetition, fairly easy to follow impressions without discernment or attention. The gangliar matter of the thalami or of the striated bodies would serve, according to Ferrier, to constitute the connection between the impression and movement in all those actions that, being voluntary at first, then became unconscious because of habit. He writes, "In these cases, we may *suppose* that the impressions made on sensory organs go towards the optic thalami, and pass from there to the striated bodies rather than going through the larger and conscious circle, that is, through the motor and sensory centers of the hemispheres."[40]

Given this, it is natural, according to the author, that these actions, being so automatically organized in the basal ganglia, would still exist even following the removal of the hemispheres. But no one, I think, would believe that an impression ends up establishing its own habitual passage through base ganglia only because it passes through the cortex repeatedly. Not even this hypothesis illuminates, therefore, but rather obscures the functioning of the mechanism of these actions. The actions performed by animals without hemispheres are also held to be unconscious, not so much because of any of their characteristics, but only because they are performed without the intervention of cortical layers: "The reaction," writes Ferrier, "between the optic thalami and the striated bodies being outside the realm of consciousness (localized in the cortical levels) is still outside the sphere of properly called psychological activity."[41] But we know that the cortical layers must be considered conscious by their very character, and we have shown above how we can distinguish them through experience from those that are due to mere excitability.[42]

We can here add that there are also other criteria to distinguish an automatic coordination from a conscious one. In the first case, although the movement depends on stimulation of the muscle fiber by means of the nerves, coordination is a fact, so to speak, which is exterior to the nervous system and depends on the arrangement in which the muscle fibers are found in the area that is set in motion. This coordination is found in the heart, the stomach, and other organs where the muscle fiber, contracting always in the same way through the stimulation received, still determines varied and coordinated movements in the organ. And no one could explain this automatic coordination by placing the seat of one faculty in the ganglia of these organs, a faculty, as Goltz would say, self-adapting. But this mechanism is lacking in conscious coordination; the so-called muscles of animal life do not present a mechanism whose architecture is organized for a purpose, and thus excitability's effects on them are resolved only in clonic or tonic contractions and the intervention of will is always necessary to organize them into a special mechanism.

We cannot say how movements that have become habitual, and to which we pay no attention, have become unconscious; nor is it our purpose to discuss them here, but we will explain it in full in the practical (that is, not theoretical) part of this study. On the other hand, Ferrier's hypothesis of an automatic organization of the voluntary movements in the basal ganglia, which is a problem in itself, does not solve other problems and must be supported by new and stranger suppositions. It is well known that this author bases his theory essentially on the fact, which he believes to be constant, that in the higher animals, such as man and monkeys, a circumscribed lesion of the cerebral cortex induces a permanent sensory and motor paralysis.[43] We can now ask why the automatic organization of the movements in the basal ganglia does not function in these animals and why it remains a privilege of only a few animals of the lower orders.

Here another hypothesis was indispensable. This happened, says Ferrier, because "Animals differ according to the degree of independence of the organization of their motor activities in the lower and mesencephalic centers."[44] But it is not understood why this difference exists. Ferrier thinks that in the higher animals, since actions are more complex, they require the will from the beginning in order to be accomplished, and thus it is training that gradually comes to perfect their strength. In lower animals, on the other hand, because will is almost nonexistent, the control and the coordination of their actions are complete from the beginning and need no effort of training. He writes, "These animals are, to a large extent, conscious automatons."[45] This is why "their cortical motor centers are of little importance and can be removed without causing disturbances in their ordinary activities."[46] Thus Ferrier finds that the animals whose hemispheres are easier to remove are those that, as soon as they are born, perform all the movements of which they are capable, such as birds that "hatch totally equipped, like Athena springing from the head of Zeus."[47] In man, for whom training is long and difficult, "automatism in itself is barely separable from the centers of consciousness and will."[48] But aside from the fact that these data are in relationship with the degree of development to which, at the moment of birth, the nervous system has arrived, a degree that varies in different orders, this author forgets that the pigeon is an animal requiring a rather long period of time to acquire all its movements; it ˙s in fact on the pigeon that the non-existent effects of hemisphere removal have usually been demonstrated. But we shall not dwell on this any longer. We believe that this, and many other difficulties, could be set aside in the same way; proceeding with this method, never before heard of in proper sciences, there will never be a fact impossible to accommodate under any theory.

Brown-Séquard's hypothesis. A hypothesis that, by considering the localization in general in the encephalon of sensitivity and will, functions better in reconciling localization with all facts presented to us by experience, is the one formulated by Brown-Séquard: "The nerve cells of the encephalon that constitute the centers controlling any specific function whatsoever, far from forming a group or a conglomeration in a distinct and well-circumscribed area, are instead spread about, so that each function has elements for this purpose in very different areas of the encephalon. Hence a localization of functions exists, but in scattered cells, which do not form, as believed, distinct aggregates either in the circumvolutions, or elsewhere."[49]

We can only oppose to this hypothesis a criticism of the concept of the function that some have thought to be localized in predetermined nerve cells and that cannot be accepted by science, as we will have occasion to prove later. [We can also point out] the difficulties that the transmission of sensory impressions and of motor stimulations on will, which we have described in preceding pages, presents. It is certain, however, that given the localization of sensitivity and movement in the encephalic organs as a general thesis, one would succeed better with this hypothesis than with the previous ones in reconciling it with results that are clearly contrary to experience. But we are satisfied with having demonstrated that no proofs of any kind exist that sensitivity and will have an exclusive seat in the nerve centers and that we are in no way obliged, regarding this issue, to maintain the concept of a transmission.

Conclusion

Summarizing the above: (1) Science maintains this concept based not on fact but on a merely speculative idea of the ancients. (2) Given that concept, we must admit within the nervous system an anatomic tendency that is contradicted by all the teachings of anatomy. (3) We must assume distinct conductive routes that go in the opposite direction from the sensory impressions and the motor impulses of will; we must support this hypothesis, which is contradicted by experience, with other hypotheses equally inconsistent. (4) There are no facts that can be used to support a proof of transmission; many of these facts cannot be explained by this concept unless we use another endless series of suppositions, which would still be contradicted by experience. We can conclude that the concept itself is false and must be absolutely rejected. However, it would still be impossible to deduce, as a practical result of this study, that sensitivity is diffused and that will determines nerve action on the spot. It is first necessary that another age-old prejudice be removed, one that impedes the understanding of these functions. This prejudice would take away equally from the physiology of the nervous system and [be] characteristic of experimental doctrine, even if the concept of double transmission is eliminated.

Reference Matter

Notes

PREFACE

1. Harvey Cushing's 1901 visit to Sherrington's Liverpool laboratory noted that a gorilla cost "over $1,000" at that time. Even in 1901 working conditions were still difficult: "Eight-hour observations in a room at 82 degrees—87 degrees. . . . Hard work. The gorilla was anaesthetized in his cage with blankets around it. We also were almost anaesthetized at the same time. Grunbaum had a revolver so that if [it] came to the worst, there would be no scandal" (Fulton 1946: 198).

2. Ferrier dedicated the book to Jackson.

3. Information here is drawn from the following sources and is more formally discussed in Chapter 3: Rawlings 1913; Holmes 1954; Ferrier 1873–1883; Sachs 1957; National Hospital Records 1870–1901.

4. Lenny Schatzman, personal communication, Fall 1978.

CHAPTER ONE

1. Some related work in this tradition that analyzes strategies, tasks, and contexts of science as part of the sociology of work can be found in the following references: on simplification and triangulation processes in science, Star 1983, 1986; on science and social worlds, Gerson 1983a; on anomalies and scientific work organization, Star and Gerson 1987; on problem substitutions in botanical work, Volberg 1983a; on recalcitrant materials and intersections in reproductive biology, Clarke 1985, 1987; and on social movements and problems in cancer research, Fujimura 1987, 1988. The work of William C. Wimsatt (such as 1980a, 1981) and James Griesemer (1983, 1984) in the philosophy of science has also called for an understanding of science based on research strategies and work contexts, as has the work of Carl Hewitt (1985), Walt Scacchi (1984), and Les Gasser (1984) in computer science.

2. Since the early nineteenth century, however, reflex physiologists had sought and found various reflex pathways through the nervous system (Fearing 1930; Liddell 1960). A research tradition that sought to link specific parts

of the anatomy with functions had begun, although it did not yet touch the cerebral hemispheres (Olmstead 1944).

3. Although primitive forms of surgery on the skull and outer parts of the brain had been attempted since earliest times, modern intracranial neurosurgery began in 1884 (Bennett and Godlee 1884; MacEwan 1893; Ballance 1922).

CHAPTER TWO

1. I agree with Julius Roth's (1974) caveat that we need historical, developmental studies that focus on working groups' interests and their conflicts and locations in society, rather than fruitless demarcation battles about what a profession is and what an occupation is.

Similarly, Donald Light's discussion (1983) of the development of professional schools in the United States points to a complex set of professionalization processes that cannot be easily characterized as the same across situations. Light states that many professional training schools are in a structurally ambiguous position because they conduct academic research and vocational training at the same time. This leads to an irregular and layered development of professional autonomy, in which clients play an extremely important part. The description of professionalization in this chapter attempts to encompass some of these complexities and ambiguities.

2. Self-regulation was in the form of prosecution of so-called quacks, licensing restrictions, and attempts to abolish competitive fee setting (Lyons 1966; Poynter 1966b).

3. Paul Starr (1982) discusses many similar events in the American context. His analysis of the "changing ecology" of medical practice and the institutional shape of the U.S. system indicates that changes such as these created similar conditions.

4. The hospital at Queen Square was founded by two women, the Chandler sisters, in 1860. The lack of medical care for a paralytic relative was the catalyst for their fund-raising effort. They raised the money for the hospital by selling hand-strung necklaces door-to-door.

CHAPTER THREE

1. It does seem, however, that this uncertainty is inescapable in basic research. As one referee for Star 1985a pointed out, the very taxonomy of uncertainty presented here is itself an example of taxonomic (if not diagnostic, technical, and political) uncertainty; I too have had to ascertain "what type of thing this is" from an array of phenomena. I have tried to resolve the un-

certainties here, however, not by converting them into unempirically testable ideal types or jettisoning individual differences, but by delineating varieties and conditions.

Wimsatt and Griesemer have already suggested an extension to this work, which is mapping the interactions between types of uncertainty (such as between diagnostic and political) under varying conditions (private communication, July 1984).

2. For general discussions of uncertainty in medical sociology, see Fox 1957; Light 1979. Little attention has been paid to varieties of uncertainty or to work-based strategies for its management, although organizational theorists have begun the analysis (such as Fiddle 1980) and several psychologists have worked on decision-making under uncertainty (for example, Tweney, Doherty, and Mynatt 1981; Kahneman, Slovic, and Tversky 1982).

For purposes of consistency, I primarily use the past tense in describing the situations faced by these investigators. I do not mean to imply that these problems no longer exist in neurology or neurosurgery; many remain unresolved (see, for example, Franklin and Doelp 1983).

3. I am grateful to William Wimsatt for pointing out several uses of such forms and to Elihu Gerson for clarifying several related issues. Muriel Bell has pointed out that it is not surprising that patients often left blanks in the seizure sheets, since seizures often lead to lapses in memory—another source of uncertainty.

4. The work in progress of H. S. Becker and associates on representations has begun to analyze such packaging in a number of fields, including statistics and the production of computer graphics (unpublished memoranda, Northwestern University 1983–84; Becker 1986). Other important work in progress points in similar directions (see Law 1985, 1987; Latour 1986).

5. James Carrier's concept of "masking" (1979) is particularly interesting in light of discussions of deletion of uncertainty.

CHAPTER FOUR

1. Fujimura's examination of contemporary cancer research organization (1986) reveals a similar pattern of problem construction via biochemical techniques and compares academic and industrial research.

2. The work of computer scientists on open systems and distributed knowledge systems in artificial intelligence is important here (see Hewitt and deJong 1984; Gasser 1987; and my discussion in Chapter 1).

3. I am grateful to Sheryl Ruzek for bringing this important point to my attention.

CHAPTER FIVE

1. For contemporary versions of this criticism see Wimsatt 1976, Laurence 1977, Glassman 1978, and Klein 1978. Laurence's discussion of the category error problem is especially interesting.

2. There is not space here to discuss this interesting facet of the debate in detail, but perhaps future research will trace this development. The work of Sherrington, for example, was strongly affected by the work of Goltz, although Sherrington transformed Goltz's ideas into a localizationist model. The themes of inhibition and dynamogenesis are familiar to generations of researchers on the nervous system—since Bernard, at least—and the history of these concepts would contain rich information on assimilation and transformation of concepts between schools or researchers with different stylistic commitments.

3. Ferrier also stated: "Out of the heterogeneous mass of cases collected by Brown-Séquard, not one, to my mind, satisfies the requirements of scientific evidence in a question of this kind. Even, however, if we did admit every one of them, the logical deduction from such facts, taken by the side of the hundreds of thousands of cases of cross paralysis, would be, not that the doctrine of the cross action of the cerebral hemisphere is untenable, but that there may be exceptions" (1876: 233). Ferrier then went on to make similar criticisms of Goltz.

4. Todes 1981 has a good discussion of this in the history of Russian psychophysiological research.

5. For a good discussion of a contemporary controversy about significance, see Morrison and Henkel 1970.

6. I would almost certainly agree with Brown-Séquard here. As discussed in Chapter 3, autopsies and postmortem examinations were often hurried and inexpert.

7. The original quote reads: "Toute la valeur des faits d'irritation de la zone dite motrice de l'écorce cérébrale, d'après les expériences de Fritsch et Hitzig, de David Ferrier, de Horsley et Beevor et tant d'autres, est certainement annulée par des expériences démontrant que la même partie d'une côté de cette zone est capable de produire, suivant les circonstances, des mouvements identiques."

CHAPTER SIX

1. An excellent summary of these positions may be found in James 1890 (pp. 128–82). A strikingly similar review of these positions may also be found in Eccles 1982, which gives essentially a point-for-point recap of the positions laid out by James.

2. At Queen Square, Jackson's prestige seems to have carried over to the present day. While researching this book there, I had to carry several of Jackson's casebooks from one room to another. A nurse in the corridor regarded me solemnly, then said in a reverent half-whisper, "Is that himself's?"

3. Later, when Laycock was at Edinburgh, David Ferrier became his student. Critchley 1960a says that Laycock influenced Ferrier to go into neurology.

4. William James attacked this view harshly, calling it sloppy thinking (1890: 134–36).

5. A similar tacit interlevel switch, with accompanying reductionism, is discussed in Wimsatt 1976. Although he does not explicitly discuss it in detail, Wimsatt also states that the source for arriving at these levels of analysis, or for confounding them, is a pragmatic need of working scientists (see especially pp. 231–32).

CHAPTER SEVEN

1. This point becomes clear if one remembers that the unit of analysis here is not human beings, but interactions. Thus the stratification of perspectives forming nature is not anthropocentric but is a formal statement about interaction that includes everything. (See Dewey 1916, 1920, 1938; Dewey et al. 1917; James 1928 [1907]; Mead 1964 [1927]; Bentley 1975a [1943].)

APPENDIX B

AUTHOR'S NOTE: It was not possible to obtain complete bibliographical information for all sources cited by Panizza. I wish to thank Linda Tucker of the Smithsonian Institution, Washington, D.C., for her assistance in locating this information.

1. Charles-Edouard Brown-Séquard, *Doctrines relatives aux principles actions des centres nerveux* (Paris: G. Masson, 1879), p. 19.

2. Pierre Flourens, *Recherches expérimentales sur les propriétés et les fonctions du système nerveux,* 2d ed. (Paris, 1842), p. 78.

3. Georges Cuvier, *Rapport sur le mémoire de Flourens. Accad. des Science de l'Istit. 22 Luglio 1822.* Cited in Flourens, op. cit., p. 78.

4. Flourens, op. cit., p. 79.

5. Cuvier, op. cit., p. 79.

6. François Achille Longet, *Traité de physiologie,* vol. II (Paris: V. Masson et Fils, 1850), Pt. II, pp. 38–39.

7. Edmond Felix Alfred Vulpian, *Leçons sur la physiologie générale et comparée du système nerveux* (Paris: Germer Baillière, 1866), p. 672.

8. Filippo Lussana and A. Lemoigne, *Fisiologia dei centri nervosi encefalici* (Padova, 1871), p. 35.

9. Vulpian, op. cit., p. 681.

10. Ibid., p. 682.

11. Ibid., p. 679.

12. These experiments were all carried out at the Rome Medical Institute in the presence of many colleagues.

13. David Ferrier, *De la localisation dans les maladies cérébrales*, trans. Henri C. de Varigny (Paris: Germer Baillière, 1879), p. 32.

14. Smoler, "Physiologie und Pathologie des Nervensystems" or "Psychiatrie," *Vierteljahrschrift für die praktische heilkunde*, BD. 79, (1863): 90–110 or 110–120.

15. Vulpian, op. cit., p. 709.

16. Armand Trousseau, see Vulpian, op. cit., p. 711.

17. Alfred Armand Louis Marie Velpeau, "Abcès symptomatique d'un nécrose du pariétal," *Lancette Française, Gazette des hôpitaux civils et militaires*, no. 39 (April 2, 1864): 153–54.

18. Vulpian, op. cit., p. 711.

19. We do not want to insist too much on [Longet's] cases, which refer to other problems in the annals of pathology. In his work, pure cases are always very rare, and are of absolutely no value in the controversy on localization.

In fact, apart from necropsy, which is always embarrassing, the phenomena that accompany a brain lesion are by some considered to be the immediate effect of the lesion and are by others considered to be indirect and accessory phenomena or phenomena of inhibition. This is up to the pathologist to decide and depends on the theory he has of the mind—the essential symptom could become the indirect symptom and vice versa, and this group of symptoms are then most subject to debate. A shining example comes from Wernicke's work. Here Meynert's anatomical ideas are accepted, as well as Hitzig and Fritsch's and Munk's physiological ones—and these stand against all who disagree with the localizationists, and are used to build his own edifice. When problems referred to by others are not attributed to typographical or printing errors or to sampling problems, he always finds a way of conciliating the facts with the theory—the presence or lack of a symptom that should be there, according to the theory, and that corresponds to a particular lesion. [Wernicke] decides which of the various symptoms should be taken as direct, and which should be indirect. He takes statistical criteria as fallacious because, they say, pure cases of organ illnesses are rare. He repudiates Nothnagel's criterion, which would take as focal symptoms only those that persist over a period beyond that of the accessory symptoms. It will be seen by this and other expedients that Wernicke can easily bring pathology into accord with anatomy and with the physiology of the localizationists.

20. Flourens, op. cit., pp. 244, 264.

21. Vulpian, op. cit., p. 708.

22. Hermann Lotze, *Principes généraux de psychologie physiologique*, trans. A. Penjon (Paris, 1876), p. 73.

23. Ferrier, op. cit., p. 410.

24. Ibid., pp. 414–15.

25. Ibid., p. 416.

26. Ibid., p. 418.

27. Ibid.

28. Ibid.

29. Ibid.

30. Ibid., p. 321.

31. Ibid., p. 410.

32. Ibid., p. 413.

33. Gustav Theodor Fritsch and Eduard Hitzig, "Über die elektrische Erregbarkeit des Grosshirns," *Archiv für anatomie, physiologie und wissenschaftliche medizin, 1870, Het. III* (Leipzig, 1870), pp. 300–332.

34. Ferrier, op. cit., pp. 322ff.

35. Ibid., p. 318.

36. Ibid., p. 400.

37. Ibid., p. 442.

38. Munk found the visual center not, like Ferrier, in the cortex, but in an extension of the occipital lobe. Tamburini and Luciani say that they got the same results in their experiments. However, in one experiment they ablated the supposed visual center according to Ferrier (in the cortex) and to Munk (occipital lobe) and found that it did not produce blindness. Localizationists interpreted these facts to mean that there were other visual centers in the lower ganglia: "Besides those in the cortex, they say, we need to posit other basal centers of vision" (Luciani and Tamburini, *Sui centri psico-sensorii corticali* [Rome: Reggio Emilia, 1879], pp. 77–78).

39. Ferrier, op. cit., pp. 66.

40. Ibid., p. 406.

41. Ibid., p. 408.

42. [See Chapter 3 in this volume, pp. 67–68.]

43. Ferrier, op. cit., p. 335.

44. Ibid., p. 404.

45. Ibid., p. 426.

46. Ibid., p. 427.

47. Ibid.

48. Ibid., p. 428.

49. Brown-Séquard, op. cit., p. 7.

References Cited

Abel-Smith, B.
  1964 *The Hospitals, 1800–1948*. London: Heinemann.
Althaus, J.
  1880 "On Some Points in the Diagnosis and Treatment of Brain Disease." *Brain* 3: 299–308.
Anderson, J.
  1966 "Medical Education and Social Change." In Poynter 1966a (pp. 207–18).
Angel, R.
  1961 "Jackson, Freud and Sherrington on the Relation of Brain and Mind." *American Journal of Psychiatry* 118: 193–97.
Ardila, A., and F. Ostrosky-Solis (eds.)
  1984 *The Right Hemisphere: Neurology and Neuropsychiatry*. New York: Gordon and Breach.
Atkins, R.
  1878 "A Case of Right Hemiplegia, Hemiaesthesia, and Aphasia, Having for Its Prominent Anatomical Lesion Softening of the Left Lateral Lobe of the Cerebellum." *Brain* 1: 410–17.
Ballance, C.
  1922 "A Glimpse into the History of the Surgery of the Brain." *The Lancet* 202: 165–72.
Barnes, B., and J. Law
  1976 "Whatever Should Be Done with Indexical Expression?" *Theory and Society* 3: 223–37.
Barnes, B., and S. Shapin (eds.)
  1979 *Natural Order: Historical Studies of Scientific Culture*. Beverly Hills: Sage.
Bartholow, R.
  1874 "Correspondence. Experiments on the Function of the Human Brain." *British Medical Journal* 1: 727.
Becker, H. S.

1960   "Notes on the Concept of Commitment." *American Journal of Sociology* 66: 32–40.

1967   "Whose Side Are We On?" *Social Problems* 14: 239–47.

1970   *Sociological Work*. Chicago: Aldine.

1982   *Art Worlds*. Berkeley: University of California Press.

1986   *Doing Things Together*. Evanston, Ill.: Northwestern U. Press.

Becker, H. S., B. Geer, E. C. Hughes, and A. L. Strauss

1961   *Boys in White: Student Culture in Medical School*. Chicago: University of Chicago Press.

Becker, P.

1983   Lecture delivered to Tremont Research Institute, San Francisco, Calif., March.

Beevor, C. E., and V. Horsley

1890   "Electrical Excitation of the So-Called Motor Cortex and Internal Capsule in an Orang-utang." *Philosophical Transactions of the Royal Society* 181: 129–58.

1894   "A Further Minute Analysis by Electric Stimulation of the So-Called Motor Region (Facial Area) of the Cortex Cerebri in the Monkey (Macacus Sinicus)." Ibid. 185: 39–81.

Benham, F. L.

1879   "Review of G. H. Lewes, *The Study of Psychology*. London: Truber, 1879." *Brain* 2: 390–400.

1880   "Review of Scientific Transcendentalism by 'D. M.' London: Williams and Norgate, 1880." *Brain* 3: 374–83.

Bennett, A. H.

1878   "Metalloscopy and Metallotherapy." *Brain* 1: 331–39.

Bennett, A. H., and R. J. Godlee

1884   "Report of Tumour Removal." *The Lancet* (Dec. 10): 1090–91.

Bentley, A.

1926   *Relativity in Man and Society*. New York: G. P. Putnam.

1975a [1954]   *Inquiry into Inquiries: Essays in Social Theory*. Ed. S. Ratner. Westport, Conn.: Greenwood Press.

1975b   "The Fiction of 'Retinal Image.'" In Bentley 1975a (pp. 268–85).

1975c   "The Human Skin: Philosophy's Last Line of Defense." In Bentley 1975a (pp. 195–211).

Benton, A.

1978   "The Interplay of Experimental and Clinical Approaches in Brain Lesion Research." In Finger 1978 (pp. 49–68).

Bijker, W., T. P. Hughes, and T. Pinch (eds.)

1987   *The Social Construction of Technological Systems: New Directions in the Sociology and History of Technology*. Cambridge, Mass.: MIT Press.

Bishop, W. J.
1960 "Hughlings Jackson (1835–1911)." *Cerebral Palsy Bulletin* 2: 3–4.
Blackwood, W.
1961 "The National Hospital, Queen Square, and the Development of Neuropathology." *World Neurology* 1: 331–35.
Blumer, H.
1969 *Symbolic Interactionism: Perspective and Method.* Englewood Cliffs, N.J.: Prentice-Hall.
Bogen, J. E., and G. M. Bogen
1976 "Wernicke's Region—Where Is It?" *Annals of the New York Academy of Sciences* 280: 834–43.
Boring, E. G.
1950 *A History of Experimental Psychology.* 2d ed. New York: Appleton-Century-Crofts.
Bosk, C.
1979 *Forgive and Remember: Managing Medical Failure.* Chicago: University of Chicago Press.
Bowker, G.
1984 "If Ever Time Was: The Social and Scientific Perception of Time in England and France in the 1830s." Ph.D. diss., University of Melbourne.
1989 "L'Industrialisation de la science." In M. Serres, ed., *Introduction aux Histoires des Sciences.* Paris: Bordas.
Brain, R.
1957 "Hughlings Jackson's Ideas of Consciousness in the Light of To-day." In *The Brain and Its Functions* (pp. 83–91). Sponsored by the Wellcome Historical Medical Library. Oxford: Blackwell.
Bramwell, B.
1888 *Intracranial Tumours.* Edinburgh: Pentland.
Brazier, M. A. B.
1959 "The Historical Development of Neurophysiology." In H. W. Magoun, ed., *Handbook of Physiology: Neurophysiology* (pp. 1–50). Washington, D.C.: American Physiological Society.
1961 *A History of the Electrical Activity of the Brain.* London: Pitman.
British Medical Journal
1881 "Dr. Ferrier's Localisations: For Whose Advantage?" *British Medical Journal* 2: 822–24.
Broca, P.
1861 "Remarques sur le siège de la faculté du langage articulé, suivies d'une observation d'aphémie." *Bull. Soc. Anat. Paris,* 2ième série, 6: 398–407. (Reprinted in English as "Remarks on the seat of the

faculty of articulate language, followed by an observation of aphemia," in von Bonin 1950 [pp. 49–72].)

1863 "Localisation des fonctions cérébrales, siège de la faculté du langage articulé." *Bull. Soc. d'Anthropologie. Paris* 4: 200–204.

Brown-Séquard, C. E.

1860 *Course of Lectures on the Physiology and Pathology of the Central Nervous System*. Philadelphia: Collins.

1873a "On the Mechanism of Production of Symptoms of Diseases of the Brain: Part 1." *Archives of Scientific and Practical Medicine* 1: 117–22.

1873b "On the Mechanism of Production of Symptoms of Diseases of the Brain: Part 2." *Archives of Scientific and Practical Medicine* 1: 251–66.

1873c "On Kinds of Hemiplegia Hitherto Unknown or Very Little Known, and on their Diagnosis with Spinal, Altern, and Cerebral Hemiplegia." *Archives of Scientific and Practical Medicine* 1: 134–42.

1879 "Quelques faits relatifs au mécanisme de production des paralysies et des anesthésies d'origine encéphalique." *Archives de Physiologie Normale et Pathologique*, 2ième série, 6: 199–200.

1890a "Preuves de l'insignifiance d'une expérience célèbre de MM. Victor Horsley et Beevor sur les centres appelés moteurs." *Archives de Physiologie Normale et Pathologique*, 5ième série, 2: 199–201.

1890b "Nombreux cas de vivisection pratiquee sur le cerveau de l'homme: Le verdict contre la doctrine des centres psychomoteurs." *Archives de Physiologie Normale et Pathologique*, 5ième série, 2: 762–73.

Brunton, T. L.

1882 "On the Position of the Motor Centres in the Brain in Regard to the Nutritive and Social Functions." *Brain* 4: 431–40.

Bucher, R.

1962 "Pathology: A Study of Social Movements in a Profession." *Social Problems* 10: 40–51.

Bucher, R., and J. Stelling

1973 "Vocabularies of Realism in Professional Socialization." *Social Science and Medicine* 7: 661–75.

Bucher, R., and A. L. Strauss

1961 "Professions in Process." *American Journal of Sociology* 66: 325–34.

Burdon-Sanderson, J.

1873–74 "Note on the Excitation of the Surface of the Cerebral Hemispheres by Induced Currents." *Proceedings of the Royal Society of London* 22: 368–70.

Busch, L.

1982 "History, Negotiation and Structure in Agricultural Research." *Urban Life* 11: 368–84.

Buzzard, T.
   1881   "Pain in the Occiput and Back of Neck." *Brain* 4: 130–32.
Calderwood, H.
   1879   *The Relations of Mind and Brain.* London: Macmillan.
Callon, M.
   1987   "Society in the Making: The Study of Technology as a Tool for
          Sociological Analysis." In Bijker, Hughes, and Pinch 1987 (pp. 83–
          110).
Callon, M., J. Law, and A. Rip
   1986   *Texts and Their Powers: Mapping the Dynamics of Science and Technol-
          ogy.* London: Macmillan.
Campbell, A. W.
   1905   *Histological Studies on the Localisation of Cerebral Function.* Cam-
          bridge, Engl.: Cambridge University Press.
Campbell, D. T., and D. W. Fiske
   1959   "Convergent and Discriminant Validation by the Multitrait-
          Multimethod Matrix." *Psychological Bulletin* 56: 81–105.
Cappie, J.
   1879   "On the Balance of Pressure Within the Skull." *Brain* 2: 373–84.
Carrier, J.
   1979   "Misrecognition and Knowledge." *Inquiry* 22: 321–42.
Clarke, A. E.
   1985   "Emergence of the Reproductive Research Enterprise: A Sociology
          of Biology, Medicine, and Agricultural Science in the United
          States, 1910–1940." Ph.D. diss., University of California, San Fran-
          cisco.
   1987   "Research Materials and Reproductive Science in the United
          States, 1910–1940." In G. Geison, ed., *Physiology in the American
          Context, 1850–1940* (pp. 323–50). Bethesda, Md.: American Phys-
          iological Society.
Collins, H. M.
   1975   "The Seven Sexes: A Study in the Sociology of a Phenomenon, or
          the Replication of Experiments in Physics." *Sociology* 9: 205–24.
   1985   *Changing Order: Replication and Induction in Scientific Practice.* Bev-
          erly Hills: Sage.
Collins, H. M., and T. Pinch
   1982   *Frames of Meaning: The Social Construction of Extraordinary Science.*
          London: Routledge and Kegan Paul.
Crichton-Browne, J.
   1872   "Cranial Injuries and Mental Diseases." *West Riding Lunatic Asylum
          Medical Reports* 1: 97–136.

1879 "On the Weight of the Brain and Its Component Parts in the Insane." *Brain* 1: 504–18; 2: 42–67.

1880 "A Plea for the Minute Study of Mania." *Brain* 3: 347–62.

Critchley, M.

1949 *Sir William Gowers, 1845–1915*. London: Heinemann.

1960a "Hughlings Jackson, the Man; and the Early Days of the National Hospital." *Proceedings of the Royal Society of Medicine* 53: 613–18.

1960b "The Contribution of Hughlings Jackson to Neurology." *Cerebral Palsy Bulletin* 2: 7–9.

Cushing, H.

1905 "The Special Field of Neurological Surgery." *Bulletin of the Johns Hopkins Hospital* 16: 77–87.

1910 "The Special Field of Neurological Surgery: Five Years Later." *Bulletin of the Johns Hopkins Hospital* 21: 325–39.

1913 "Realinements in Greater Medicine: Their Effect on Surgery and the Influence of Surgery upon Them." *British Medical Journal* 2: 290–97.

1920 "The Special Field of Neurological Surgery After Another Interval." *Archives of Neurology and Psychiatry* 4: 603–37.

1935 "Psychiatrists, Neurologists and the Neurosurgeon." *Yale Journal of Biology and Medicine* 7: 191–207.

Dainton, C.

1961 *The Story of England's Hospitals*. London: Museum Press.

Danziger, K.

1982 "Mid-Nineteenth Century British Psycho-physiology: A Neglected Chapter in the History of Psychology." In W. R. Woodward and M. G. Ash, eds., *The Problematic Science: Psychology in Nineteenth Century Thought* (pp. 119–46). New York: Praeger.

Daston, L.

1978 "British Responses to Psycho-physiology, 1860–1900." *Isis* 69: 192–208.

Davis. F.

1956 "Definitions of Time and Recovery in Paralytic Polio Convalescence." *American Journal of Sociology* 61: 582–87.

deWatteville, A.

1881 "Review of 'Maladies de la Moelle' by A. Vulpian. Paris: Octave Doin, 1881." *Brain* 3: 516–28.

Dewey, J.

1916 *Essays in Experimental Logic*. Chicago: University of Chicago Press.

1920 *Reconstruction in Philosophy*. New York: Henry Holt.

1929 *The Quest for Certainty: A Study of the Relation of Knowledge and Action.* New York: Minton, Balch.

1938 *Logic: The Theory of Inquiry.* New York: Holt, Rinehart and Winston.

1981 [1896] "The Reflex Arc Concept in Psychology." In J.J. McDermott, ed., *The Philosophy of John Dewey* (pp. 136–48). Chicago: University of Chicago Press.

Dewey, J., and A. Bentley

1949 *Knowing and the Known.* Boston: Beacon.

Dewey, J., A.W. Moore, H.C. Brown, G.H. Mead, B.H. Bode, H.W. Stuart, J.H. Tufts, and H.M. Kallen

1917 *Creative Intelligence: Essays in the Pragmatic Attitude.* New York: Henry Holt.

Dodds, W.J.

1877–78 "On the Localisation of the Functions of the Brain: Being an Historical and Critical Analysis of the Question." *Journal of Anatomy and Physiology* 12: 340–63, 454–93.

Duncan, J.

1879 "Clinical Cases of Hernia Cerebri." *Brain* 1: 413–17.

Duret, H.

1878 "On the Role of the Dura Mater and Its Nerves in Cerebral Traumatism." *Brain* 1: 29–47.

Eccles, J. (ed.)

1982 *Mind and Brain: The Many-Faceted Problem.* New York: Paragon House.

Edelman, G., and V. Mountcastle

1978 *The Mindful Brain: Cortical Organization and the Group-Selective Theory of Higher Brain Function.* Cambridge, Mass.: MIT Press.

Ellis, J.R.

1966 "The Growth of Science and the Reform of the Curriculum." In Poynter 1966a (pp. 155–68).

Engelhardt, H.T.

1972 "John Hughlings Jackson and the Concept of Cerebral Localization." Thesis for the M.D. degree, Tulane University.

1975 "John Hughlings Jackson and the Mind-Body Relation." *Bulletin of the History of Medicine* 49: 137–51.

Evans, A.D., and L.G.R. Howard

1936 *The Romance of the British Voluntary Hospital Movement.* London: Hutchinson.

Fearing, F.

1930 *Reflex Action: A Study in the History of Physiological Psychology*. Baltimore, Md.: Williams and Wilkins.

Ferrier, D.

1873 Experimental Researches in Cerebral Physiology and Pathology." *West Riding Lunatic Asylum Medical Reports* 3: 30–96.

1873–74 "The Localisation of Function in the Brain." *Proceedings of the Royal Society* 22: 229.

1873–1883 Unpublished laboratory notebooks, 1873–1883. Library of the Royal College of Physicians, London. MS 246/1–19.

1876 *The Functions of the Brain*. London: Smith, Elder.

1878a "Review of H. Munk, 'Weitere Mittheilungen zur Physiologie der Grosshirnrinde.' *Verhandel. der physiolog. gesselch. zu Berlin*, 9 and 10 (April 12, 1878)." *Brain* 1: 230–31.

1878b *The Localisation of Cerebral Disease*. London: Smith, Elder.

1878c "Review of H. Duret, 'Etudes Expérimentales sur les Traumatismes Cérébraux' (Versailles, 1878)." *Brain* 1: 101–10.

1879 "Pain in the Head in Connection with Cerebral Disease." *Brain* 1: 467–83.

1880 "Review of 'Animal Magnetism, Physiological Observations' by R. Heidenhain. London: Kegan Paul, 1880." *Brain* 3: 385–95.

1881 "Cerebral Amblyopia and Hemiopia." *Brain* 3: 456–77.

1882 "The Brain of a Criminal Lunatic." *Brain* 5: 62–73.

1889 "Cerebral Localization in Its Practical Relations." *Brain* 12: 36–58.

1890 *The Croonian Lectures on Cerebral Localisation*. London: Smith, Elder.

1910 "The Regional Diagnosis of Cerebral Disease." In C. Allbutt and H. D. Rolleston, eds., *A System of Medicine. Vol. VIII: Diseases of the Brain and Mental Diseases* (pp. 37–162). 2d ed. London: Macmillan.

Fiddle, S. (ed.)

1980 *Uncertainty: Behavioral and Social Dimensions*. New York: Praeger.

Finger, S. (ed.)

1978 *Recovery from Brain Damage: Research and Theory*. New York: Plenum.

Fleck, L.

1979 [1935] *Genesis and Development of a Scientific Fact*. Chicago: University of Chicago Press.

Foster, M.

1877 *A Text-Book of Physiology*. London: Macmillan.

Fox, R. C.
  1957 "Training for Uncertainty." In R. K. Merton, G. Reader, and P. Kendall, eds., *The Student-Physician* (pp. 207–41). Cambridge, Mass.: Harvard University Press.

Franklin, J., and A. Doelp
  1983 *Not Quite a Miracle: Brain Surgeons and Their Patients on the Frontier of Medicine.* New York: Doubleday.

Fraser, D.
  1881 "On Hemiplegia and Hemianaesthesia in an Idiot Boy, as the Result of Paralysis of the Left Cerebral Hemisphere, Following a Blow on the Head." *Brain* 3: 536–41.

Freidson, E.
  1968 "The Impurity of Professional Authority." In H. Becker, B. Geer, D. Riesman, and R. Weiss, eds., *Institutions and the Person* (pp. 25–34). Chicago: Aldine.

  1970a *Professional Dominance: The Social Structure of Medical Care.* New York: Atherton.

  1970b *The Profession of Medicine.* New York: Harper and Row.

French, R. D.
  1975 *Antivivisection and Medical Science in Victorian Society.* Princeton, N.J.: Princeton University Press.

Fritsch, G., and E. Hitzig
  1950 [1870] "On the Electrical Excitability of the Cerebrum." In von Bonin 1950 (pp. 73–95).

Fujimura, J.
  1986 "The Social Construction of Scientific Knowledge: A Case Study of the Molecular Genetic Bandwagon in Cancer Research." Ph.D. diss., University of California, Berkeley.

  1987 "The Social Construction of Do-able Problems in Cancer Research: Articulating Alignment." *Social Studies of Science* 17: 257–93.

  1988 "The Molecular Biological Bandwagon in Cancer Research: Where Social Worlds Meet." *Social Problems* 35: 261–83.

Fujimura, J. H., S. L. Star, and E. M. Gerson
  1987 "Méthodes de recherche en sociologie des sciences: Travail, pragmatisme et interactionnisme symbolique." *Cahiers de Recherche Sociologique* 5: 65–85.

Fulton, J. F.
  1946 *Harvey Cushing: A Biography.* Springfield, Ill.: Charles Thomas.

Fuster, J. M.
  1980 *The Prefrontal Cortex: Anatomy, Physiology and Neuropsychology of the Frontal Lobe.* New York: Raven.

Garfinkel, H.
　1967　*Studies in Ethnomethodology*. Englewood Cliffs, N.J.: Prentice-Hall.
Garfinkel, H., M. Lynch, and E. Livingston
　1981　"The Work of Discovering Science Construed with Materials from the Optically Discovered Pulsar." *Philosophy of Social Sciences* 11: 131–58.
Gasser, L.
　1984　"The Social Dynamics of Routine Computer Use in Complex Organizations." Ph.D. diss., Department of Information and Computer Science, University of California, Irvine.
　1986　"The Integration of Computing and Routine Work." *ACM Transactions on Office Information Systems* 4: 205–25.
　1987　"Distribution and Coordination of Tasks Among Intelligent Agents." Paper presented to the First Scandinavian Conference on Artificial Intelligence, Tromsö, Norway.
Geison, G.
　1972　"Social and Institutional Factors in the Stagnancy of English Physiology, 1840–1870." *Bulletin of the History of Medicine* 46: 30–58.
　1977　"Divided We Stand: Physiologists and Clinicians in the American Context." In M. J. Vogel and C. E. Rosenberg, eds., *The Therapeutic Revolution: Essays in the Social History of American Medicine* (pp. 67–90). Philadelphia: University of Pennsylvania Press.
　1978　*Michael Foster and the Cambridge School of Physiology: The Scientific Enterprise in Late Victorian Society*. Princeton, N.J.: Princeton University Press.
Gerson, E. M.
　1976　"On 'Quality of Life.'" *American Sociological Review* 41: 793–806.
　1983a　"Scientific Work and Social Worlds." *Knowledge* 4: 357–77.
　1983b　"Styles of Scientific Work and the Population Realignment in Biology, 1880–1925." Paper presented to the Conference on History and Philosophy of Biology, Granville, Ohio.
Gerson, E. M., and S. L. Star
　1986　"Analyzing Due Process in the Workplace." *ACM Transactions on Office Information Systems* 4: 257–70.
Geschwind, N., and A. Galaburda
　1987　*Cerebral Localization: Biological Mechanisms, Associations, and Pathology*. Cambridge, Mass.: MIT Press.
Glaser, B. G., and A. L. Strauss
　1964　"The Social Loss of Dying Patients." *American Journal of Nursing* 64: 119–21.

Glassman, R. B.
   1978   "The Logic of the Lesion Experiment and Its Role in the Neural
           Sciences." In Finger 1978 (pp. 3–30).
Godlee, R. J.
   1917   *Lord Lister*. London: Macmillan.
Goltz, F.
   1881   *Uber die Verrichtungen des Grosshirns*. Bonn: Strauss.
   1950 [1888]   "On the Functions of the Hemispheres." In von Bonin 1950
           (pp. 118–58).
Gould, S. J.
   1981   *The Mismeasure of Man*. New York: Norton.
Gowers, W. R.
   1878   "The Brain in Congenital Absence of One Hand." *Brain* 1: 388–90.
   1885   *Lectures on the Diagnosis of Diseases of the Brain*. London: Churchill.
Greenblatt, S. H.
   1970   "Hughlings Jackson's First Encounter with the Work of Paul Broca:
           The Physiological and Philosophical Background." *Bulletin of the
           History of Medicine* 46: 555–70.
   1972   "Some Philosophical and Clinical Background to Sherrington's
           Concept of Integrative Action." *Proceedings of the Twenty-third In-
           ternational Congress of the History of Medicine* 1: 58–61.
Griesemer, J.
   1983   "Communication and Scientific Change: An Analysis of Concep-
           tual Maps in the Macroevolution Controversy." Ph.D. diss., Uni-
           versity of Chicago.
   1984   "Presentations and the Status of Theories." *PSA 1984* 1: 337–44.
Griesemer, J., and M. Wade
   1988   "Laboratory Models, Causal Explanation and Group Selection."
           Biology and Philosophy 3: 67–96.
Head, H.
   1926   *Aphasia and Kindred Disorders of Speech*. 2 vols. New York: Macmil-
           lan.
Heelan, P.
   1977   "The Nature of Clinical Science." *Journal of Medicine and Philosophy*
           2: 20–32.
Henig, R. M.
   1981   *The Myth of Senility: Misconceptions About the Brain and Aging*. New
           York: Anchor/Doubleday.
Hewitt, C.
   1985   "The Challenge of Open Systems." *BYTE* 10: 223–42.

1986   "Offices Are Open Systems." *ACM Transactions on Office Information Systems* 4: 271–87.

Hewitt, C., and P. deJong

1984   "Open Systems." In M. L. Brodie, J. Mylopoulous, and J. W. Schmidt, eds., *On Conceptual Modeling* (pp. 147–64). New York: Springer-Verlag.

Hobson, J. M.

1882   "A Case of Tumour in the Medulla Oblongata and Pons Varolii, with Remarkable Paralytic Symptoms." *Brain* 4: 531–39.

Holmes, G.

1954   *The National Hospital, Queen Square*. Edinburgh: Livingstone.

Holton, G.

1973   *Thematic Origins of Scientific Thought*. Cambridge, Mass.: Harvard University Press.

Hornstein, G., and S. L. Star

Forthcoming   "Universality Biases: How Theories About Human Nature Succeed." *Philosophy of the Social Sciences*.

Horrax, G.

1952   *Neurosurgery: An Historical Sketch*. Springfield, Ill.: Charles Thomas.

Horsley, V.

1884   "On Substitution as a Means of Restoring Nerve Function Considered with Reference to Cerebral Localisation." *The Lancet* (July 5, 1884): 7–10.

1891   *The Structures and Function of the Brain and Spinal Cord*. London: Griffin.

1904   Casebook, 1904. Archives of the Thane Library, University College, London. MS/UNOF 12/1–2.

1906   "On the Technique of Operations on the Central Nervous System." *British Medical Journal* 3: 411–23.

Hougland, J. G., and J. M. Shepard

1980   "Organizational and Individual Responses to Environmental Uncertainty." In Fiddle 1980 (pp. 102–19).

Hubbard, R., and M. Lowe (eds.)

1979   *Genes and Gender: II, Pitfalls in Research on Sex and Gender*. New York: Gordian.

Hughes, E. C.

1966   "The Social Significance of Professionalization." In H. M. Vollmer and D. L. Mills, eds., *Professionalization* (pp. 64–70). Englewood Cliffs, N.J.: Prentice-Hall.

1971a   *The Sociological Eye*. Chicago: Aldine.

1971b "Going Concerns: The Study of American Institutions." In *The Sociological Eye* (pp. 52–64). Chicago: Aldine.

Hull, D. L.

1976 "Are Species Really Individuals?" *Systematic Zoology* 25: 174–91.

1982 "Exemplars and Scientific Change." *PSA 1982* 2: 479–503.

Hunter, R. A., and L. J. Hurwitz

1961 "The Case Notes of the National Hospital for the Paralysed and Epileptic, Queen Square, London, before 1900." *Journal of Neurology, Neurosurgery and Psychiatry* 24: 187–94.

Huxley, T.

1904 [1874] "On the Hypothesis That Animals Are Automata, and Its History." In *Method and Results, Essays* (pp. 199–250). New York: Appleton.

Ireland, W.

1879 "Review of 'The Relations of Mind and Brain' by H. Calderwood. London: Macmillan, 1879." *Brain* 1: 535–40.

Jackson, J. H.

1873a "On the Anatomical and Physiological Localisation of Movements in the Brain." *The (London) Lancet*, no. 4 (April): 197–201 [Part 1]; no. 5 (May): 245–48 [Part 2].

1873b "Observations on the Localisation of Movements in the Cerebral Hemispheres, as Revealed by Cases of Convulsion, Chorea and 'Aphasia.'" *West Riding Lunatic Asylum Medical Reports* 3: 175–95.

1875 "A Lecture on Softening of the Brain." *The (London) Lancet*, no. 11 (November): 489–94.

1876 "On Epilepsies and on the After-Effects of Epileptic Discharges." *West Riding Lunatic Asylum Medical Reports* 6: 266–309.

1878 "On Affectations of Speech from Disease of the Brain (Part 1)." *Brain* 1:304–30.

1879 "On Affectations of Speech from Disease of the Brain (Part 2)." *Brain* 2: 323–56.

1925 *Neurological Fragments with "Biographical Memoir" by James Taylor and "Recollections" by J. Hutchinson and C. Mercier.* London: Humphrey Milford.

1931 "On the Anatomical and Physiological Localisation of Movements in the Brain [revised]." In J. Taylor, ed., *Selected Writings*, Vol. 1 (pp. 37–76). London: Hodder and Stoughton.

1932a [1884] "Evolution and Dissolution of the Nervous System." In J. Taylor, ed., *Selected Writings*, Vol. 2 (pp. 45–75). London: Hodder and Stoughton.

1932b [1868–69] "Notes on the Physiology and Pathology of the Nervous System." In J. Taylor, ed., *Selected Writings*, Vol. 2 (pp. 215–37). London: Hodder and Stoughton.

1932c [1874]   "On the Nature of the Duality of the Brain." In J. Taylor, ed., *Selected Writings*, Vol. 2 (pp. 129–45). London: Hodder and Stoughton.

1932d [1887]   "Remarks on Evolution and Dissolution of the Nervous System." In J. Taylor, ed., *Selected Writings*, Vol. 2 (pp. 92–118). London: Hodder and Stoughton.

1932e [1882]   "Some Implications of Dissolution." In J. Taylor, ed., *Selected Writings*, Vol. 2 (pp. 29–44). London: Hodder and Stoughton.

1932f [1893]   "Words and Other Symbols in Mentation." In J. Taylor, ed., *Selected Writings*, Vol. 2 (pp. 205–12). London: Hodder and Stoughton.

James, A.
1881   "The Reflex Inhibitory Centre Theory." *Brain* 4: 287–302.

James, W.
1890   *The Principles of Psychology*. 2 vols. New York: Henry Holt.
1928 [1907]   *Pragmatism: A New Name for Some Old Ways of Thinking*. New York: Longmans, Green.

Jefferson, G.
1955   "Variations on a Neurological Theme—Cortical Localization." *British Medical Journal* 4: 1405–8.
1960   "Sir Victor Horsley." In *Selected Papers* (pp. 130–69). Springfield, Ill.: Charles Thomas.

Jones, C.
1946   "Some Founders of British Neurology." *New Zealand Medical Journal* 2: 143–54.

Jones, E.
1899   Class notes from 1899 class with Risien Russell (of Queen Square), at University College Hospital. MS/UNOF/14/1–2, Thane Library, University College Hospital, London.
1959   *Free Associations*. London: Hogarth.

Kahneman, D., P. Slovic, and A. Tversky (eds.)
1982   *Judgment Under Uncertainty: Heuristics and Biases*. Cambridge, Engl.: Cambridge University Press.

Kellogg, R.
1981   "Historical Perspectives." In T. F. Hornbeim, ed., *Regulation of Breathing, Part I* (pp. 3–66). New York: Marcel Dekker.

Kertesz, A. (ed.)
1983   *Localization in Neurophysiology*. New York: Academic Press.

King, L. S.
   1982 *Medical Thinking: A Historical Preface*. Princeton, N.J.: Princeton University Press.
Kinsbourne, M. (ed.)
   1978 *Asymmetrical Functions of the Brain*. Cambridge, Engl.: Cambridge University Press.
Klapp, O.
   1964 *Symbolic Leaders*. Chicago: Aldine.
Klein, B.
   1978 "The Role of Psychology in Functional Localization Research." *PSA 1978* 1: 119–33.
Klein, E., J. N. Langley, and E. A. Schafer
   1883–84 "On the Cortical Areas Removed from the Brain of a Dog, and from the Brain of a Monkey." *Journal of Physiology* 4: 231–326.
Kling, R., and E. M. Gerson
   1977 "The Social Dynamics of Technical Innovation in the Computing World." *Symbolic Interaction* 1: 132–46.
   1978 "Patterns of Segmentation and Intersection in the Computing World." *Symbolic Interaction* 1: 24–43.
Kling, R., and W. Scacchi
   1982 "The Web of Computing: Computing Technology as Social Organization." *Advances in Computers* 21: 3–78.
Knapp, P. C., and E. H. Bradford
   1889 "A Case of Tumor of the Brain; Removal; Death." *Boston Medical and Surgical Journal* 120: 325–30, 353–59, 378–81, 386–88, 439.
Knorr-Cetina, K.
   1981 *The Manufacture of Knowledge: An Essay on the Constructivist and Contextual Nature of Science*. Oxford: Pergamon Press.
Kuhn, T.
   1970 *The Structure of Scientific Revolutions*. 2d ed. Chicago: University of Chicago Press.
Lakatos, I., and A. Musgrave (eds.)
   1970 *Criticism and the Growth of Knowledge*. Cambridge, Engl.: Cambridge University Press.
Langley, J. N.
   1883–84 "The Structure of the Dog's Brain." *Journal of Physiology* 4: 248–86.
Lasagna, L.
   1972 "The Nature of Evidence." In J. D. Cooper, ed., *The Philosophy of Evidence. Vol. 3: Philosophy and Technology of Drug Assessment* (pp. 5–

24). Washington, D.C.: The Interdisciplinary Communication Associates.

Lashley, K.
1929 *Brain Mechanisms and Intelligence*. Chicago: University of Chicago Press.

Lassek, A. M.
1970 *The Unique Legacy of Doctor Hughlings Jackson*. Springfield, Ill.: Charles Thomas.

Latour, B.
1980 "Is It Possible to Reconstruct the Research Process? Sociology of a Brain Peptide." In K. D. Knorr, R. Krohn, and R. D. Whitley, eds., *The Social Process of Scientific Investigation, Sociology of the Sciences Yearbook 4* (pp. 53–73). Dordrecht: Reidel.
1986 "Visualization and Cognition." *Knowledge and Society* 6: 1–40.
1987 *Science in Action*. Cambridge, Mass.: Harvard University Press.
1988 *The Pasteurization of French Society*. Cambridge, Mass.: Harvard University Press.

Latour, B., and F. Bastide
1986 "Writing Science—Fact and Fiction." In Callon, Law, and Rip 1986 (pp. 51–66).

Latour, B., and S. Woolgar
1979 *Laboratory Life*. Beverly Hills: Sage.

Laudan, L.
1981 "William Whewell on the Consilience of Inductions." In *Science and Hypothesis* (pp. 163–80). Dordrecht: Reidel.

Laurence, S.
1977 "Localization and Recovery of Function in the Central Nervous System." Ph.D diss., Clark University.

Lave, J.
1988 *Cognition in Practice*. Cambridge, Engl.: Cambridge University Press.

Law, J.
1985 "Les textes et leurs alliés." *Culture Technique* 14: 59–69.
1986 "Laboratories and Texts." In Callon, Law, and Rip 1986 (pp. 35–50).
1987 "Technology and Heterogeneous Engineering: The Case of the Portuguese Expansion." In Bijker, Hughes, and Pinch 1987 (pp. 111–34).

Laycock, T.
1857 *Lectures on the Principles and Methods of Medical Observation and Research*. Philadelphia: Blanchard and Lea.

LeDoux, J.

1983 "Cerebral Asymmetry and the Integrated Functions of the Brain." In Young 1983 (pp. 203–16).

Levin, M.

1960 "The Mind-Brain Problem and Hughlings Jackson's Doctrine of Concomitance." *American Journal of Psychiatry* 116: 718–22.

Levins, R.

1966 "The Strategy of Model Building in Population Biology." *American Scientist* 54: 21–31.

Lewis, B.

1878a "On the Comparative Structure of the Cortex Cerebri." *Brain* 1: 79–96.

1878b "Application of Freezing Methods to the Microscopic Examination of the Brain." *Brain* 1: 348–59.

1880 "Methods of Preparing, Demonstrating and Examining Cerebral Structure in Health and Disease." *Brain* 3: 314–36.

Liddell, E. G. T.

1960 *The Discovery of Reflexes*. Oxford: Clarendon.

Light, D. W.

1979 "Uncertainty and Control in Professional Training." *Journal of Health and Social Behavior* 6: 141–51.

1983 "The Development of Professional Schools in America." In K. H. Jarausch, ed., *The Transformation of Higher Learning, 1860–1930*. Chicago: University of Chicago Press.

Lilienfeld, A.

1982 "*Ceteris paribus*: The Evolution of the Clinical Trial." *Bulletin of the History of Medicine* 56: 1–18.

Little, E. M.

1932 *History of the British Medical Association, 1832–1932*. London: British Medical Association.

Lynch, M.

1982 "'Turning up Signs' in Neurobehavioral Diagnosis." Paper delivered to the American Sociological Association, San Francisco, Calif.

1985 *Art and Artefact in Scientific Research*. London: Routledge and Kegan Paul.

Lyons, J. B.

1965 "Correspondence Between Sir William Gowers and Sir Victor Horsley." *Medical History* 9: 260–67.

1966 *Citizen Surgeon*. London: Dawnay.

MacCormac, W.

1880 *Antiseptic Surgery*. London: Smith, Elder.

MacCormac, W. (ed.)
  1881   *Transactions of the International Medical Congress*. 4 vols. London: Kolckmann.
MacEwan, W.
  1893   *Pyogenic Infective Diseases of the Brain and Spinal Cord*. Glasgow: Maclehose, 1893.
  1922   "Brain Surgery." *British Medical Journal* 2: 155–65.
MacKay, D. M.
  1978   "Selves and Brains." *Neuroscience* 3: 599–606.
MacKenzie, S.
  1878   "Embolic Hemiplegia with Optic Neuritis." *Brain* 1: 400–409.
Manier, E.
  1986   "Social Dimensions of the Mind / Body Problem: Turbulence in the Flow of Scientific Information." *Science and Technology Studies* 4: 16–28.
Marks, H. M.
  1984   "Ideas as Social Reforms: The Legacies of Randomized Clinical Trials." Unpublished manuscript, Harvard Medical School.
Maudsley, H.
  1890   *Body and Mind: An Enquiry into Their Connection and Mutual Influence, Specially in Reference to Mental Disorders*. 2d ed. New York: Appleton.
McClelland, J. L., D. Rumelhart, and G. E. Hinton
  1986   "The Appeal of the PDP." In Rumelhart, McClelland, and the PDP Research Group 1986 (pp. 3–44).
McClelland, J.L., D. Rumelhart, and the PDP Research Group
  1986   *Parallel Distributed Processing: Exploration in the Microstructure of Cognition*. Vol. 2: *Psychological and Biological Models*. Cambridge, Mass.: MIT Press.
McEachron, D. L.
  1986   *Functional Mapping in Biology, Medicine, Computer Assisted Autoradiography*. Experimental Biology and Medicine: Monographs in Interdisciplinary Topics, vol. 2. Basel: Karger.
McGill University
  1936   *Neurological Biographies and Addresses*. London: Oxford / Humphrey Milford.
McMenemey, W. H.
  1966   "Education and the Medical Reform Movement." In Poynter 1966a (pp. 135–54).

Mead, G. H.
   1917 "Scientific Method and the Individual Thinker." In Dewey et al.
         1917 (pp. 176–227).
   1964 [1927] "The Objective Reality of Perspectives." In A. J. Reck, ed.,
         Selected Writings (pp. 306–19). Chicago: University of Chicago
         Press.
Meehl, P. E.
   1977 "Specific Etiology and Other Forms of Strong Inference: Some
         Quantitative Meanings." *Journal of Medicine and Philosophy* 2: 33–53.
Merritt, H. H.
   1975 "The Development of Neurology in the Past 50 Years." In *Centen-
         nial Anniversary Volume of the American Neurological Association* (pp.
         3–10). New York: Springer.
Mills, K.
   1879 "Five Cases of Disease of the Brain, Studied Chiefly with Reference
         to Localisation." *Brain* 1: 547–68.
Mitchell, E. G.
   1960 "Writings of Hughlings Jackson." *Cerebral Palsy Bulletin* 2: 34–35.
Morgenstern, O.
   1963 *On the Accuracy of Economic Observations.* Princeton, N.J.: Princeton
         University Press.
Morrison, D. E., and R. E. Henkel (eds.)
   1970 *The Significance Test Controversy.* Chicago: Aldine.
Murphy, E. A.
   1977 "Classification and Its Alternatives." In H. T. Engelhardt, S. F.
         Spicker, and B. Towers, eds., *Clinical Judgement: A Critical Ap-
         praisal.* Dordrecht: Reidel.
   1982 "Analysis and Interpretation of Experiments." *Journal of Medicine
         and Philosophy* 7: 307–25.
National Hospital Records
   1870–1901 Unpublished hospital case records (casebooks), formerly of
         the National Hospital for the Paralysed and Epileptic, Queen
         Square, London. Archives of the National Hospital for Nervous
         Diseases, London.
Newman, C.
   1957 *The Evolution of Medical Education in the Nineteenth Century.* Ox-
         ford: Oxford University Press.
   1966 "The Rise of Specialism and Postgraduate Education." In Poynter
         1966a (pp. 169–93).

Olmstead, J. M. D.

    1944   "Historical Note on the *noeud vital* or Respiratory Center." *Bulletin of the History of Medicine* 16: 343.

    1946   *Charles-Edouard Brown-Séquard: A Nineteenth Century Neurologist and Endocrinologist*. Baltimore, Md.: Johns Hopkins University Press.

O'Neil, W. M.

    1985   "Associationism." In Adam Kuper and Jessica Kuper, eds., *The Social Science Encyclopedia* (p. 48). London: Routledge and Kegan Paul.

Orne, M. T.

    1962   "On the Social Psychology of the Psychological Experiment: With Particular Reference to Demand Characteristics and Their Implications." In R. Rosenthal and R. Rosnow, eds., *Artifact in Behavioral Research* (pp. 143–79). New York: Academic Press.

Paget, S.

    1919   *Sir Victor Horsley: A Study of His Life and Work*. London: Constable.

Panizza, M.

    1887   *La fisiologia de sistema nervoso e i fatti psichici*. 3d ed. Rome: Manzoni.

Parry, N., and J. Parry

    1976   *The Rise of the Medical Profession: A Study of Collective Social Mobility*. London: Croom Helm.

Pauly, P. J.

    1984   "The Appearance of Academic Biology in Late-Nineteenth-Century America." *Journal of the History of Biology* 17: 369–97.

Peacock, A.

    1982   "The Relationship Between the Soul and the Brain." In F. C. Rose and W. F. Bynum, eds., *Historical Aspects of the Neurosciences* (pp. 83–98). New York: Raven.

Penfield, W., and L. Roberts

    1959   *Speech and Brain Mechanisms*. Princeton, N.J.: Princeton University Press.

Peterson, M. J.

    1978   *The Medical Profession in Mid-Victorian London*. Berkeley: University of California Press.

Pinch, T. J.

    1980   "Theoreticians and the Production of Experimental Anomaly: The Case of Solar Neutrinos." In K. D. Knorr and R. Krohn, eds., *The Social Process of Scientific Investigation*. Vol. 4 (pp. 77–106). Dordrecht: Reidel.

1981 "The Sun-Set: The Presentation of Certainty in Scientific Life." *Social Studies of Science* 11: 155.

Pinker, R.
1966 *English Hospital Statistics, 1861–1938.* London: Heinemann.

Polanyi, M.
1964 *Personal Knowledge: Towards a Post-Critical Philosophy.* New York: Harper and Row.

Popper, K., and J. Eccles
1977 *The Self and Its Brain: An Argument for Interactionism.* Berlin: Springer International.

Pound, R.
1967 *Harley Street.* London: Michael Joseph.

Poynter, F. N. L. (ed.)
1966a *The Evolution of Medical Education in Britain.* London: Pitman.
1966b "Education and the General Medical Council." In Poynter 1966a (pp. 195–205).

Rabagliati, A.
1878a "Review of 'Three Cases of Softening of the Brain in the Left Hemisphere, Affecting the Ascending Frontal Convolution or the Anterior Marginal' by Ugo Palmerini (Siena), d'Archivio Italiano per le Malattie Nervose, Sept. and Nov. 1877." *Brain* 1: 424–31.
1878b "Review of 'Clinical Researchers on the Motor Centres of the Limbs,' *Journal de Therapeutique,* 1877." *Brain* 1: n.p.
1879 "Review of the work on localization of Luciani and Tamburini." *Brain* 1: 529–44.
1882 "Review of 'The Physiology of the Nervous System in Its Relation to Psychic Facts' by M. Panizza (La Fisiologia de Sistema Nervosa nelle sue Relazioni coi Fatti Psichici). Rome: Manzoni." *Brain* 5: 105–9.

Raichler, M. E.
1982 "Positron Emission Tomography." In Thompson and Green 1982 (pp. 145–56).

Rainger, R., K. R. Benson, and J. Maienschein (eds.)
1988 *The American Development of Biology.* Philadelphia: University of Pennsylvania Press.

Rasmussen, T.
1982 "Localizational Aspects of Epileptic Seizure Phenomena." In Thompson and Green 1982 (pp. 177–203).

Rawlings, B. B.
1913 *A Hospital in the Making.* London: Pitman.

Reader, W. J.
  1966 *Professional Men: The Rise of the Professional Classes in Nineteenth-Century England.* London: Weidenfeld and Nicolson.
Reichardt, W. E., and T. Poggio
  1981 *Theoretical Approaches in Neurobiology.* Cambridge, Mass.: MIT Press.
Reiser, S. J.
  1978 *Medicine and the Reign of Technology.* Cambridge, Engl.: Cambridge University Press.
Restivo, S.
  1983 *The Social Relations of Physics, Mysticism and Mathematics.* Boston: D. Reidel.
  1984 "Representation and the Sociology of Mathematical Knowledge." In B. Schiele and C. Belisle, eds., *Les Savoirs dans les Pratiques Quotidiennes.* Paris: CNRS.
Richards, R.
  1982 "Darwin and the Biologizing of Moral Behavior." In W. R. Woodward and M. G. Ash, eds., *The Problematic Science: Psychology in Nineteenth Century Thought* (pp. 85–115). New York: Praeger.
Riese, W.
  1959 *A History of Neurology.* New York: M.D. Publications.
  1977 *Selected Papers on the History of Aphasia.* Amsterdam: Swets and Zeritlinger.
Roberts, R. S.
  1966 "Medical Education and the Medical Corporation." In Poynter 1966a (pp. 69–88).
Rogers, L.
  1930 "The History of Craniotomy." *Annals of Medical History* 2: 495–514.
Role, A.
  1977 *La vie étrange d'un grand savant: Le professeur Brown-Séquard.* Paris: Plon.
Rolleston, G.
  1874 Referee's Report of the Royal Society, May 12, 1874. Unpublished MS, Archives of the Royal Society.
Rosen, G.
  1968 *Madness in Society.* New York: Harper and Row.
Rosenberg, C.
  1976 *No Other Gods: On Science and American Social Thought.* Baltimore: Johns Hopkins University Press.

Rosenthal, R.
 1963 "On the Social Psychology of the Psychological Experiment: The Experimenter's Hypothesis as Unintended Determinant of Experimental Results." *American Scientist* 51: 268–83.
 1966 *Experimenter Effects in Behavioral Research*. New York: Appleton-Century-Crofts.
Ross, J.
 1882a "Review of 'Studien über das Bewusstsein; Studien über die Sprachvorstellungen; Studien über die Bewegungsvorstellungen,' by S. Stricker (Wien, 1879–1882, pamphlets, no pub. data given)." *Brain* 5: 99–105.
 1882b "Labio-glosso-pharyngeal Paralysis of Cerebral Origin." *Brain* 5: 145–69.
Roth, J.
 1974 "Professionalism: The Sociologist's Decoy." *Sociology of Work and Occupations* 1: 6–23.
Rothschuh, K.
 1973 *History of Physiology*. Huntington, N.Y.: Krieger.
Rudwick, M.
 1985 *The Great Devonian Controversy*. Oxford: Oxford University Press.
Rumelhart, D., and J. L. McClelland
 1986 "PDP Models and General Issues in Cognitive Science." In McClelland, Rumelhart, and the PDP Research Group 1986 (pp. 110–46).
Rumelhart, D., J. L. McClelland, and the PDP Research Group
 1986 *Parallel Distributed Processing: Explorations in the Microstructure of Cognition*. Vol. 1: *Foundations*. Cambridge, Mass.: MIT Press.
Rumelhart, D., P. Smolensky, J. L. McClelland, and G. E. Hinton
 1986 "Schemata and Sequential Thought Processes in PDP Models." In McClelland, Rumelhart, and the PDP Research Group 1986 (pp. 7–57).
Ryle, G.
 1949 *The Concept of Mind*. New York: Barnes and Noble.
Sachs, E.
 1952 *The History and Development of Neurological Surgery*. New York: Paul Hoeber.
 1957 "Reminiscences of an American student." *British Medical Journal* 1: 916–17.
Scacchi, W.
 1984 "Managing Software Engineering Projects: A Social Analysis." *IEEE Transactions on Software Engineering* SE-10: 49–59.

Schafer, E. A.
    1883–84 "Report on the Lesions, Primary and Secondary, in the Brain
            and Spinal Cord of the Macacque Monkey Exhibited by Profs. Fer-
            rier and Yeo." *Journal of Physiology* 4: 316–26.
Schiller, F.
    1979 *Paul Broca: Founder of Anthropology, Explorer of the Brain*. Berkeley:
            University of California Press.
    1982 "Neurology: The Electrical Root." In F. C. Rose and W. F. Bynum,
            eds., *Historical Aspects of the Neurosciences* (pp. 1–11). New York:
            Raven.
Schmitt, F. O.
    1979 "The Role of Structural, Electrical, and Chemical Circuitry in Brain
            Function." In Schmitt and Worden 1979 (pp. 1–40).
Schmitt, F. O., and F. Worden (eds.)
    1979 *The Neurosciences: Fourth Study Program*. Cambridge, Mass.: MIT
            Press.
Seguin, E.
    1881 "A Second Contribution to the Study of Localized Cerebral Le-
            sions." *Journal of Nervous and Mental Disease* 8: 510–52.
Sejnowski, T. J.
    1986 "Open Questions About Computation in Cerebral Cortex." In
            Rumelhart, McClelland, and the PDP Research Group 1986 (pp.
            372–89).
Shapin, S.
    1979 "Homo Phrenologicus: Anthropological Perspectives on an His-
            torical Problem." In Barnes and Shapin 1979 (pp. 41–71).
Shapter, L.
    1880 "On Functional Athetosis and Incoordination of Movement."
            Brain 3: 402–7.
Sharpey-Schafer, E.
    1927 *History of the Physiological Society During Its First Fifty Years, 1876–
            1926*. London: Cambridge University Press.
Sherrington, C. S.
    1906 *The Integrative Action of the Nervous System*. New York: Charles
            Scribner's.
Shortliffe, E. H.
    1976 *Computer-Based Medical Consultations: MYCIN*. New York: Elsev-
            ier.
Simmel, G.
    1903–4 "The Sociology of Conflict." *American Journal of Sociology* 9:
            490–501.

Simon, H.

1973 "The Structure of Ill-Structured Problems." *Artificial Intelligence* 4: 181–201.

1981 *The Sciences of the Artificial.* Cambridge, Mass.: MIT Press.

Smart, J. J. C.

1955 "Spatialising Time." *Mind* 64: 239–41.

Smith, C. U. M.

1982 "Evolution and the Problem of Mind: Part II. John Hughlings Jackson." *Journal of the History of Biology* 15: 241–62.

Smith, H. W.

1959 "The Biology of Consciousness." In C. M. Brooks and P. F. Cranefield, eds., *The Historical Development of Physiological Thought* (pp. 2–3). New York: Hafner.

Sperry, R. W.

1980 "Mind-Brain Interaction: Mentalism, Yes; Dualism, No." *Neuroscience* 5: 195–206.

Spillane, J. D.

1981 *The Doctrine of the Nerves: Chapters in the History of Neurology.* Oxford: Oxford University Press.

Stanley, J. P., and S. W. Robbins

1977 "Secret Agents and Truncated Passives." *Forum Linguisticum* 2: 33–46.

Star, S. L.

1982 "Terminology as a Map of Segmentations and Intersections in Scientific Work." Paper presented to the International Sociological Association, Mexico City.

1983 "Simplification and Scientific Work: An Example from Neuroscience Research." *Social Studies of Science* 13: 205–28.

1985a "Scientific Work and Uncertainty." *Social Studies of Science* 15: 391–427.

1985b "Epistemological Revolutions Are Not Made of Words." *Contemporary Sociology* 14: 315–18.

1986 "Triangulating Clinical and Basic Research: British Localizationists, 1870–1906." *History of Science*, 24: 29–48.

1988a "The Structure of Ill-Structured Solutions: Boundary Objects and Heterogeneous Distributed Problem Solving." Paper presented to the Eighth AAAI Conference on Distributed Artificial Intelligence, Lake Arrowhead. Technical Report, Department of Computer Science, University of Southern California.

1988b "Introduction: The Sociology of Science and Technology." *Social Problems* 35: 197–205.

Star, S. L., and E. M. Gerson
  1987 "The Management and Dynamics of Anomalies in Scientific Work." *Sociological Quarterly* 28: 147–69.
Starr, P.
  1982 *The Social Transformation of American Medicine*. New York: Basic.
Strauss, A. L.
  1961 *Images of the American City*. New York: Free Press.
  1978a "A Social World Perspective." *Studies in Symbolic Interaction* 1: 119–28.
  1978b *Negotiations*. San Francisco: Jossey-Bass.
Strauss, A. L. (ed.)
  1979 *Where Medicine Fails*. New Brunswick, N.J.: Transaction.
Strauss, A. L., L. Schatzman, R. Bucher, D. Ehrlich, and M. Sabshin
  1964 *Psychiatric Ideologies and Institutions*. New York: Free Press of Glencoe.
Swazey, J.
  1969 *Reflexes and Motor Integration: Sherrington's Concept of Integrative Action*. Cambridge, Mass.: Harvard University Press.
  1970 "Action Propre and Action Commune: The Localization of Cerebral Function." *Journal of the History of Biology* 3: 213–34.
Temkin, O.
  1945 *The Falling Sickness: A History of Epilepsy from the Greeks to the Beginnings of Modern Neurology*. Baltimore: Johns Hopkins University Press.
Thompson, R. A., and J. R. Green (eds.)
  1982 *New Perspectives in Cerebral Localization*. New York: Raven.
Thorwald, J.
  1959 *The Triumph of Surgery*. New York: Pantheon.
Tizard, B.
  1959 "Theories of Brain Localization from Flourens to Lashley." *Medical History* 3: 132–45.
Todes, D. P.
  1981 "From Radicalism to Scientific Convention: Biological Psychology in Russia from Sechenov to Pavlov." Ph.D diss., University of Pennsylvania.
Toulmin, S.
  1976 "On the Nature of the Physician's Understanding." *Journal of Medicine and Philosophy* 1: 32–50.
Tucker, R. C. (ed.)
  1978 *Karl Marx and Frederick Engels: The Marx-Engels Reader*. 2d ed. New York: Norton.

United States Surgeon-General's Office
    1919 *Manual of Neurosurgery*. Washington, D.C.: Government Printing Office.
University College Hospital, London
    1880–1890 "Minutes of the Medical Society." Unpublished manuscript.
Urquhart, A. R.
    1878 "Cases of Cerebral Excitement Treated by Mustard Baths." *Brain* 1: 126–27.
    1880 "Cortical Lesions of the Cerebral Hemispheres." *Brain* 3: 430–32.
Vaughan, H. G.
    1975 "Psychosurgery and Brain Stimulation in Historical Perspective." In W. Gaylin, J. S. Meister, and R. C. Neville, eds., *Operating on the Mind* (pp. 24–72). New York: Basic.
Viets, H. R.
    1938 "West Riding, 1871–1876." *Bulletin of the History of Medicine* 6: 477–87.
Volberg, R.
    1983a "Commitments and Constraints: The Development of Ecology in the United States, 1900–1940." Ph.D diss., University of California, San Francisco.
    1983b "Use and Abuse of the 'Species' Concept in Biology." Paper presented to the Conference on History and Philosophy of Biology, Granville, Ohio.
von Bonin, G. (ed.)
    1950 *Some Papers on the Cerebral Cortex*. Springfield, Ill.: Charles Thomas.
Walker, A. E.
    1957 "The Development of the Concept of Cerebral Localization in the Nineteenth Century." *Bulletin of the History of Medicine* 31: 99–121.
Waller, A.
    1882 "N. Buboff and R. Heidenhain on Phenomena of Excitation and Inhibition in the Cerebral Motor Centres." *Brain* 5: 138–40.
Walshe, F. M. R.
    1947 *On the Contribution of Clinical Study to the Physiology of the Cerebral Motor Cortex*. Edinburgh: Livingstone.
    1957 "Some Reflections upon the Opening Phase of the Physiology of the Cerebral Cortex, 1850–1900." In *The Brain and Its Functions* (pp. 223–34). Sponsored by the Wellcome Historical Medical Library. Oxford: Blackwell.
    1961 "Contributions of John Hughlings Jackson to Neurology." *Archives of Neurology* 5: 119–31.

Warren, H. C.
  1921   *A History of the Association Psychology*. London: Constable.
West Riding Pauper Lunatic Asylum
  1871–74   *Reports of the West Riding Pauper Lunatic Asylum, 1871–74*.
Whewell, W.
  1967 [1847]   *The Philosophy of the Inductive Sciences*. Vol. 2. London: Frank
       Cass.
Williams, R., and J. Law
  1980   "Beyond the Bounds of Credibility." *Fundamenta Scientiae* 1: 295–
       315.
Wimsatt, W. C.
  1976   "Reductionism, Levels of Organization, and the Mind-Body Prob-
       lem." In G. Globus, G. Maxwell, and I. Savodnik, eds., *Consciousness
       and the Brain: A Scientific and Philosophical Inquiry* (pp. 199–267).
       New York: Plenum.
  1980a "Reductionist Research Strategies and Their Biases in the Units of
       Selection Controversy." In T. Nickles, ed., *Scientific Discovery: Case
       Studies* (pp. 213–59). Dordrecht: Reidel.
  1980b "Randomness and Perceived-Randomness in Evolutionary Biol-
       ogy." *Synthese* 43: 287–329.
  1981   "Robustness, reliability, and overdetermination." In M. B. Brewer
       and B. E. Collins, eds., *Scientific Inquiry and the Social Sciences* (pp.
       124–62). San Francisco: Jossey-Bass.
  1986   "Developmental Constraints, Generative Entrenchment, and the
       Innate-Acquired Distinction." In P. W. Bechtel, ed., *Integrating Sci-
       entific Disciplines* (pp. 185–208). Dordrecht: Martinus-Nijhoff.
Witelson, S.
  1983   "Bumps on the Brain: Right-Left Asymmetry as a Key to Func-
       tional Lateralization." In S. Segalowitz, ed., *Language Functions and
       Brain Organization* (pp. 117–44). New York: Academic Press.
Woolgar, S.
  1980   "Discovery, Logic and Sequence in a Scientific Text." In K. D.
       Knorr, R. Krohn, and R. Whitley, eds., *The Social Process of Scientific
       Investigation*. Vol. 4 (pp. 239–68). Dordrecht: Reidel.
  1981   "Interests and Explanations in the Social Study of Science." *Social
       Studies of Science* 11: 365–94.
Wynne, B.
  1979   "Physics and Psychics: Science, Symbolic Action and Social Con-
       trol in Late Victorian England." In Barnes and Shapin 1979 (pp.
       167–84).

Yeo, J. B.
    1878   "A Case of Large Tumour of the Left Cerebral Hemisphere, with
           Remarkable Remissions in the Symptoms." *Brain* 1: 273–76.
Young, A. W. (ed.)
    1983   *Functions of the Right Cerebral Hemisphere*. New York: Academic
           Press.
Young, R. M.
    1970   *Mind, Brain and Adaptation in the Nineteenth Century: Cerebral Lo-
           calization and Its Biological Context from Gall to Ferrier*. Oxford: Clar-
           endon.
Zenzen, M., and S. Restivo
    1982   "The Mysterious Morphology of Immiscible Liquids: A Study of
           Scientific Practice." *Social Science Information* 21: 447–73.

Name Index

Abel-Smith, Brian, 47, 52
Althaus, Julius, 142
Ardila, Alfredo, 183
Atkins, Ringrose, 71, 138

Baillarger, 223
Bain, Alexander, 17, 159
Bastian, Charlton, 57
Becker, Howard S., 235
Becker, Peter, 24
Beevor, Charles Edward, 84, 152–53, 180, 236
Bell, Muriel, 235
Bennett, Hughes, 14, 58–59, 71, 139
Bentley, Arthur F., 19, 116, 157–58
Bernard, Claude, 54, 122, 236
Bogen, G. M., 67
Bogen, Joseph, 67
Boring, E. G., 159
Bowker, Geoffrey, 31
Bradford, E. H., 91, 99
Broca, Paul, 1, 5, 11, 142
Brown-Séquard, Charles-Edouard, 5–7, 61, 122–25 *passim*, 130–32, 136–53 *passim*, 164, 184, 215, 228, 236
Bucher, Rue, 39, 88
Bucknill, John C., 32
Burdon-Sanderson, John, 53, 55, 57, 146
Busch, Lawrence, 39
Buzzard, Thomas, 74

Campbell, Alfred W., 103, 105
Campbell, Donald, 108
Cappie, James, 167
Carpenter, William B., 217
Carrier, James, 235
Carville, 221
Chandler sisters, 234

Charcot, Jean-Martin, 105
Clarke, Adele, 31, 39, 233
Collins, Harry, 190–91
Crichton-Browne, James, 31, 49, 81, 106
Critchley, Malcolm, 236
Cushing, Harvey, 79
Cuvier, Georges, 216–17

Darwin, Charles, 8, 55, 57, 195
Descartes, René, 9, 156
Dewey, John, 62, 175
Dodds, 141, 170, 176
Duret, 146, 221

Eccles, John, 236
Engelhardt, H. Tristam, Jr., 160, 172
Engels, Friedrich, 16

Ferrier, David, 5, 7, 31, 32, 48, 49, 55–57, 58, 59, 67, 71, 72, 77, 82–85, 90, 97–107 *passim*, 122, 124, 129–53 *passim*, 159, 168, 170, 175, 179, 180, 200–201, 203, 205–6, 210, 221–28, 233, 236, 239
Fiske, D. W., 108
Flourens, Pierre, 4, 11, 128, 135, 200–202, 216, 220–21
Foster, Michael, 53, 55–56, 80, 146, 151, 195
Fox, Renée, 235
Freidson, Eliot, 111
French, Richard, 54
Freud, Sigmund, 175
Fritsch, Gustav, 5, 13, 100, 124, 129, 142–43, 146, 153, 199–201, 223, 236, 238
Fujimura, Joan Hideko, 39, 88, 233, 235
Fuster, Joaquin, 182

Galaburda, Albert, 184–85

Gall, Franz Joseph, 16, 220, 223, 224
Gasser, Les, 233
Geison, Gerald, 54, 104, 110
Gerson, Elihu, 233, 235
Geschwind, Norman, 184–85
Godlee, Rickman, 14–15, 58–59, 99, 139
Golgi, Camillo, 127
Goltz, Friedrich, 55–56, 61, 104–5, 106,
    122–32 *passim*, 136–37, 141, 142, 144,
    148–49, 150, 154, 199–214, 218–19, 227,
    236
Gowers, William, 14, 48, 69, 74, 76, 78,
    99, 105, 139, 149–50, 169–70, 175
Griesemer, James, 112, 233, 235

Head, Henry, 85, 165
Heelan, Patrick, 109
Henkel, R. E., 236
Hewitt, Carl, 20–21, 233
Hitzig, Eduard, 5, 13, 85, 100, 124, 129,
    142–43, 146, 153, 199–209 *passim*, 223,
    236, 238
Hooker, Joseph, 55
Horsley, Victor, 14, 52, 57, 60, 68–79 *pas-*
    sim, 84, 88–89, 90–91, 97–103 *passim*,
    114, 121, 122, 131–39 *passim*, 152–53, 175,
    180, 184, 236
Hughes, Everett C., 28, 41
Huxley, Thomas Henry, 8, 55, 57, 172

Jackson, John Hughlings, 5, 31, 32, 48,
    50, 55, 57–58, 59, 67, 72, 97, 100–101,
    122, 142–43, 147–77 *passim*, 183, 184,
    233, 236
James, William, 119, 123–24, 236, 237
Jones, Ernest, 89

Kertesz, Andrew, 185
King, Lester, 109–10
Klapp, Orren, 162
Kling, Rob, 39
Knapp, Philip Coombs, 91, 99
Kuhn, Thomas, 17, 64

Lashley, Karl, 28
Latour, Bruno, 31, 61, 64, 116, 120, 190
Laurence, Scott, 236
Lave, Jean, 28
Law, John, 191
Laycock, Thomas, 164, 236

LeDoux, Joseph, 183
Lemoigne, 217
Levins, Richard, 21, 24
Lewes, G. H., 167–68
Lewis, Bevan, 31
Light, Donald, 234, 235
Lister, Lord Joseph, 14
Longet, 217, 220–21, 238
Lotze, Hermann, 222
Luciani, Luigi, 83, 123, 124, 146,
    239
Ludwig, Carl, 54
Lussana, 217
Lynch, Michael, 64, 191

MacCormac, Sir William, 59
MacEwan, William, 101
Magendie, François, 102–3
Manier, Edward, 191
Marks, Harry, 110
Marshall, T. H., 41
Marx, Karl, 16
Maudsley, Henry, 169
McClelland, James, 186–87
McEwan, William, 101
Mead, George Herbert, 16, 24
Meynert, 238
Morgenstern, Oskar, 109
Morrison, D. E., 236
Munk, Hermann, 83, 124, 201–9 *passim*,
    238, 239
Murphy, Edmond, 110

Nothnagel, 238

Ostrosky-Solis, Feggy, 183

Paget, Stephen, 68, 121
Panizza, Mario, 123, 125, 129–30, 141–42,
    214–29
Parry, Jose, 47
Parry, Noel, 47
Pasteur, Louis, 60, 120
Pauly, Philip, 31
Pavlov, Ivan, 29
Peacock, Andrew, 8, 177–78
Penfield, Wilder, 180–81
Peterson, Mildred, 44
Pinch, Trevor, 110, 190–91

Rabagliati, A., 83

Ramon y Cajal, Santiago, 127
Rasmussen, Theodore, 183
Rawlings, Burford, 57, 85
Roberts, Lamar, 181
Rolleston, George, 55, 90
Rosenberg, Charles, 31
Roth, Julius, 234
Rudwick, Martin, 127
Rumelhart, David, 186–87
Ruzek, Sheryl, 235

Scacchi, Walt, 233
Schafer, Edward A. *See* Sharpey-Schafer,
    Edward
Schmitt, F. O., 28
Sechenov, I., 29
Sejnowski, Terrence, 187
Semon, Felix, 75
Shäfer, Edward A. *See* Sharpey-Schafer,
    Edward
Sharpey-Schafer, Edward, 25, 53, 55, 57,
    105, 195
Sherrington, Charles Scott, 4, 6–8, 28,
    97, 154, 176–78, 190–91, 233, 236
Simmel, Georg, 118, 121
Simon, Herbert, 93, 189
Smoler, 219, 224
Spencer, Herbert, 5, 57, 58, 159, 165, 173
Spillane, John D., 76, 89
Spurzheim, Johann, 16
Star, Susan Leigh, 233
Starr, Paul, 234

Steinem, Gloria, 163
Stelling, Joan, 88
Strauss, Anselm, 39, 110, 163, 174, 196
Swazey, Judith, 4

Tamburini, Augusto, 83, 123, 146, 239
Taylor, James, 58
Tempkin, Owsei, 100–101
Tizard, Barbara, 4
Todes, Daniel, 29, 196–97, 236
Toulmin, Stephen, 110
Trousseau, 220

Velpeau, 220
Volberg, Rachel, 93
von Bergmann, Ernst, 90
Vulpian, 217–18, 220–21

Wade, Michael, 112
Wallace, Russell, 57
Walshe, F. M. R., 7
Wernicke, 238
Whewell, William, 108
Wimsatt, William C., 24, 109, 235, 237
Witelson, Sandra, 183, 184
Woolgar, Steve, 64, 109
Wynne, Brian, 191

Yeo, Gerald, 56, 71, 132
Young, Andrew, 183
Young, Robert M., 159

Subject Index

Ablation (of cerebral cortex), 15, 148–49, 200–201, 205–6, 210–11, 214
Abstraction, 111–12
Action at a distance, 122, 131, 148
Acute illness, 49–51
Allies, enrollment of, 61
Anesthetic, 60
Anomalies, 8, 22, 33–34, 94–95, 106, 107, 112–13, 114, 142, 149, 185, 188, 191, 194, 204; absorption of, 25–26, 63–64, 130, 153–54; "anomaly bows," 134; and debate about localization, 120; of inconstant correlation between function and region, 6, 84–85, 125–26, 130–32, 169, 175, 177, 202, 214–15, 219–21, 227–28; jettisoning, 68, 71, 84, 87, 113; management of, 35, 145; and paradigms, 17, 63–64
Antilocalizationism, 43, 60–61, 106–7. *See also* Diffusionist theories
Antisepsis, 14, 59–60, 83, 84, 99–100, 158
Antivivisection, 13, 25, 80–81, 111, 162, 165, 194; and British physiology, 26, 40–42, 55–57, 80; and licensing, 70; and localizationism, 106; and trial of Ferrier, 56–57; and uncertainty, 68, 70
Aphasia, 68, 74, 90, 159–60, 166, 171, 183, 185
Articulation work, 110
Artifacts, 64–65. *See also* Anomalies
Artifacts in localization research, 64, 82, 83, 84, 113; diffusion of current, 69, 84, 146–47; surgical side effects, 69, 83
Artificial intelligence, 20, 285
Association psychology, 16–17, 27, 132, 159
Asylums, 12, 26, 31–32, 49–50

Atlases of the brain. *See* Maps of the brain
Atomism, 127
Automata theory, 185
Autopsy, 11, 12, 31, 70–71, 74, 81, 102, 103, 140, 148, 150, 236

Bandwagons, 23
Basic research: and evidence, 96, 99–101, 104–6. *See also* Triangulation
Blindness, 74, 201–7 *passim*, 212
Brain, 32, 49, 81, 146, 151, 167
Brain lesions, 12
Brain surgery. *See* Surgery, brain
Brain tumors. *See* Tumors, brain
Brain waves. *See* EEGs
Brain weight, 12
British Medical Association, 41, 56
British Medical Journal, 145
Broca's area. *See* Speech area
Building block theories (of mind), 166, 169–70

Cartesian dualism. *See* Psychophysical parallelism
Cerebral cortex, 79, 100, 122, 137, 182, 183, 187, 239; ablation of, 104, 200–214; electrical stimulation of, 5, 13, 69, 82–84, 101, 102, 128, 129, 146, 152, 157, 180, 185, 199–200, 223; mapping, 71, 84, 89–90, 97, 152–53; motor centers, 143, 180, 203, 206, 217–18, 223; and vision, 202–3, 207–12 *passim*, 223
Chloroform, 60, 83
Chronic illness, 50–51, 112, 182
Classification (of diseases). *See* Uncertainty; Taxonomies, clinical
Clinical evidence, 80, 96–106 *passim*,

110–11, 115, 179–81. *See also* Triangulation
Clinical trials, 134
Coherence, 21, 95, 191
Coincident boundaries, 157, 194–95
Collège de France, 122
Commitments, 22, 24
Complications, 112–13
Computer science, 185, 186, 189
Concomitance, doctrine of, 160–61, 165–72 *passim*. *See also* Psychophysical parallelism
Connectionism, 28, 182, 186–87
Consciousness, 169–76 *passim*, 181, 225, 226, 227–28
Contralateralization, 138, 142
Cruelty to Animals Act (1876), 55–56, 70, 106
Cumulative reification, 133. *See also* Reification
Cybernetics, 28

Debates, scientific, 98, 118–21, 125, 127–28, 191; Ferrier-Goltz debate, 55–56, 104–5, 106; modes of, 152–53; *ad hominem* arguments, 153; and triangulation, 98; tacit, 152–53; about localization, 9, 27, 55–56, 92–93, 118–54, 161
Debating tactics, 132–51, 194; *ad hominem* arguments, 133, 141–43, 153, 194; appeal to status quo, 133, 151; compiling credibility, 138–40; control of focus, 145–51; referencing the unknown, 147–50; and diplomacy, 134–37; hierarchies of credibility, appeal to, 143–44; hierarchies of credibility, manipulation of, 140–44; "more scientific than thou," 140–42; organizational, 144–45; truisms, 135–36, 141, 144
Deficiency diseases, 68, 74
Definition of the situation, 16, 30
Depression, 173
Diagnosis, 45, 164; of brain tumors, 59, 99; and taxonomies, 109–10, 113, 145, 150, 191, 195
Diffusionist theories, 4, 6, 28, 60–61, 70, 119, 121–24; of Brown-Séquard, 5–7, 122, 123, 125, 130–31, 137, 138, 139, 228; of

Goltz, 55, 125, 136–37, 199–214; of Lashley, 28; of Panizza, 123, 125, 129–30, 214–29; of Sherrington, 7–8. *See also* Debates, scientific
Dissolution, theory of, 165, 171. *See also* Spencer, Herbert
"Doability" (of a scientific problem), 39, 188
Doctors, house and staff, 47–49
Dualism, 158. *See also* Psychophysical parallelism
Dynamogenesis, 122, 236

Edinburgh University, 236
EEGs (electroencephalograms), 14, 35, 128
Engineering, 93
Epilepsy, 31, 52, 53, 179, 195; seizures, 52, 68, 70, 71, 74, 100, 157, 164, 181, 183; and Brown-Séquard, 122; forms of, 69, 99–100; and Jackson, 50, 97, 100–101, 121, 164–66, 183; "march" of symptoms, 5, 72, 112; social aspects of, 69; treatments for, 40–41, 53, 76
Epileptics, 1, 26, 166, 182
ESP (extrasensory perception), 190–91
Evolutionary biology, 141, 162, 182, 183, 193, 194; and alliance with localizationism, 8, 26, 55, 141, 195; Darwinian, 175; Spencerian, 5, 57–58, 159, 165, 171–73
Exemplary cases, 15, 50, 72–73, 85, 139
Experimenter expectations, 134
Experiments, 11–12, 69, 82–84, 102–3, 124–25; animal experiments, 49, 82, 104–5, 106, 114, 122–23, 150, 201; natural experiments, 11, 101, 102, 103, 196; regulation of, 55–56; vivisection, 14–15. *See also* Antivivisection
Expert systems, 110

Faculties, 217
Frozen accidents, 24–25
Functions of the Brain, The, 84, 103, 168

Garbage categories. *See* Residual categories
Generalization, 34, 65
General Medical Council, 44
Generative entrenchment, 192

Germ theory of disease, 158

Hemiplegia, 105, 143, 206, 224
Hemispheric asymmetry, 183–84, 186,
    224
Hierarchical organization of nervous
    system, 194, 196
Hierarchy of credibility, 23, 116–17
Histology, 15, 103
Holism, 127
Hospital for Epilepsy and Paralysis,
    Oxford, 81
Hospitals, English: admissions, 51, 79–
    80; charity, 10, 42, 52; funding of, 42,
    46, 48–49, 51, 80; specialist, 46–49,
    124; voluntary, 46, 47–49, 52
Human nature, 148
Hysteria, 173

Idealism, 176
Ideal types, 68, 71, 87, 89–91, 111–12,
    114
Ill-structured problems, 189–90
Incompleteness, of scientific theories, 62,
    192, 193
Individual differences, 67, 73, 82, 87, 89,
    98, 111, 114
Individualism, 158, 176
Inertia, 22, 23, 133, 192, 196
Inhibition, 122, 137, 151, 236, 238
Inscriptions, 19
Inseparability of parts (of a scientific
    theory), 192, 194
*Integrative Action of the Nervous System,
    The*, 4, 6, 97, 176
Intelligence, 206–17 *passim*, 221
Interests, 17–18
Internalist vs. externalist, 17, 197
International Medical Congress (1881),
    55, 56, 80, 104, 150, 193

King's College, London, 210

Lancet, The, 58
Lead poisoning, 68, 74
Learning disabilities, 182
Lesions, 12, 13, 68, 122, 130, 141, 148, 149,
    173, 183, 185, 227
Licensing, medical, 44
Localization: failures of, 83, 85, 90–91,

99–102, 105, 126; of tumors, 14, 15, 99,
    136
Localizationists: collegial networks, 58,
    81
Localization theory: assumptions of, 9,
    175–76; debate about, 9, 27, 55–56, 92–
    93, 118–54, 161; defined, 4; diagnosis
    using, 58, 59; institutional base of, 38–
    61; legacy of, 27–28, 175–98; vs. diffu-
    sionist theory, 4; public perception
    of, 87, 106–7, 120, 201
"Logic of deletion," 12, 103, 132, 151, 152,
    175, 180
London Galvanic Hospital, 48

Maps of the brain, 3, 4, 8, 14, 15, 63, 67,
    71, 89–90, 100, 114–15, 125, 152
Medical education, 41, 42, 45; in hospi-
    tals, 46–47, 164 193, 234
Medical reform, 41–44 *passim*, 124, 192
Medical Reform Act (1858), 44–45
Medical technology, 26, 40–41, 58–60,
    82, 188
Memory, 169–70, 179
Mental illness, 50
Mind, 63, 77–78, 119, 158, 168–69, 170,
    172, 182–88 *passim*
Mind/brain relationship, 3, 9, 121, 155–
    56, 162, 166, 175, 178–79, 193. *See also*
    Psychophysical parallelism
Mistakes, 33–34
Momentum, 23, 133, 192, 193
Montreal Neurological Institute, 179

National Hospital for Nervous Diseases,
    Queen Square, London. *See* National
    Hospital for the Paralysed and Epilep-
    tic, Queen Square, London
National Hospital for the Paralysed and
    Epileptic, Queen Square, London, 3,
    10, 15, 36, 38, 40–41, 51, 57, 68, 77, 78,
    79–80, 89, 98, 112, 149–50, 196, 236;
    and brain surgery, 70; and epilepsy,
    53; founding of, 234; as specialist hos-
    pital, 42, 46, 48–49
Necessary connections, 25
Neurasthenia, 68, 173
Neurology, 10, 59, 75–76, 77–79, 99, 102,
    113, 157, 163, 179
Neuropsychiatry, 178–81

Neuropsychology, 185
Neurosciences, 180–87
Neurosurgery, 59, 70, 79, 97–100, 178–81
Normal science, 64
Nursing, 42, 49, 78

Open systems, 19–21, 26, 188, 192, 235
Ophthalmology, 75, 76
Optic neuritis, 76

Paradigm, 17, 23, 63, 64, 65, 94
Parallel distributed processing, 186–87. *See also* Connectionism
Paralysis, 13, 31, 52, 68, 74, 137, 141, 157, 215, 216
Pathognomonic sign, 75–76
Pathology, 10, 15, 99, 100, 102, 113, 157, 214
Patients, 42, 49, 51–53, 59–60, 72, 119–20, 174; in asylums, 26, 31, 32; as subjects, 26, 32, 42, 46, 101–2, 104–5
Perspectives, 16, 18, 94–95, 116
PET (positron emission tomography) scans, 181, 182, 184
Phrenology, 4, 16, 43, 223, 224
Physicians: consulting, 47–49; house, 78
Physiological experiments, 69, 82, 141
Physiological Society, 26, 55, 56, 81, 165
Physiology, 10, 32, 53–58, 80, 101, 103, 111, 113, 157, 162, 195; anatomical approach in English, 53–54, 104, 113; institutional base of English, 54, 56–57, 103–4, 194; and uncertainty, 103–4
Plasticity, 21–22, 191
Plausible bridges, 162, 166–73. *See also* Psychophysical parallelism
Postmortem evidence, 10. *See also* Autopsy
Potassium bromide, 53, 76
Pragmatism, 123
Principles of Psychology, 123
Profession, 88, 234; defined, 41–42; and scientific theories, 39
Professionalization, 39; of medicine, 41–46, 234
Psychiatry, 162, 179
Psychoanalysis, 94
Psychology, 179, 216–17
Psychophysical parallelism, 9, 27, 78, 155–77 *passim*, 186, 188, 193, 194–95

Psychosurgery, 27, 179–80

Quacks, medical, 44
Queen Square. *See* National Hospital for the Paralysed and Epileptic, Queen Square, London

Rabies, 60
Racism, 197
Recovery of function, 68, 126, 201, 205–6, 220, 221; and substitution, 6, 126, 224
Reductionism, 158, 237
Redundancy, 126, 131
Reflexes, 210; integration of, 176–78; reflex physiology, 166, 169, 233–34; reflex tests, 10, 52, 75
Reification, 24, 64, 192, 193–94
Relativism, 29–30
Reliability, 107–8. *See also* Robustness
Replication, 190–91
Representations, 235
Representation theories, 166–67, 170–73, 177, 184
Residual categories, 173–74
Robustness, 18–19, 21, 24, 107–11, 133, 192
Royal College of Physicians, 173
Royal Society, 55, 90
Russian neurophysiology, 28, 29, 196, 236

Satisficing, 93
Scientific knowledge: as heterogeneous, 20–21, 62, 116
Scientific materials, 67, 81, 91; animals, 69, 71, 82, 83, 84, 106, 114, 150, 210–14, 233; brains, 32, 70, 71; cadavers, 70, 81; and uncertainty, 70, 99
Scientific practice. *See* Work
Scientific theories, 25, 97; as collective, 18, 40, 61; decentralized nature of, 24, 27, 62, 92, 115–16, 117; incompleteness of, 19, 23, 24, 62, 115; and pluralism, 24; reification of, 24; as work, 14–19, 34, 60
Seizures, 74, 100, 114, 122. *See also* Epilepsy
Senility, 173
Sepsis, 99, 113
Sexism, 197

Side effects, 73
Simplification, 23, 33, 35, 65, 188–91
Skin, 157–58
Skull, 157
Social worlds, 163, 233
Specialist hospitals, 46–49, 124
Specialization, medical, 40, 43, 45–47,
    51, 68, 77, 193
Speech area, 4, 5, 11, 12, 105, 129, 181, 183
Standardization, 72
St. Bartholomew's Hospital, 48
Stroke, 68, 139
Stylistic conflicts in science, 126–28, 131–
    32, 144, 147, 236
Substrata (of mind/brain), 166, 168, 172,
    180, 182, 184, 194
Surgeons: and physicians, 80; status of,
    41, 77–78, 80, 236
Surgery, brain, 10, 14–15, 57, 58, 59–60,
    73–74, 78–79, 81, 99–102, 113, 114, 121,
    139, 157, 158, 179, 195, 234; attitudes
    toward, 78–79, 100; failures of, 88–89,
    90–91, 99; and first localizationist
    operation, 14, 99; complications of, 14
Symbolic interactionism, 3, 233
Symbolic leader: Jackson as, 162–66
Symptoms, 52, 68–69, 72, 100, 105
Syphilis, 31, 68, 74, 100

Taxonomies, clinical, 52, 75, 92, 109–10,
    113, 150
Treatments, 75, 76, 79, 141, 176
Trephining, 79, 143
Triangulation, 26–27, 34, 65, 81, 88, 89,
    132, 156–57, 158, 161, 191; defined, 96;
    and inertia, 192; of methods, 107–8; of
    researchers, 107; and uncertainty, 97

Truth, 18, 19, 21, 38
Tuberculosis, 68, 100
Tumors, brain, 59, 68–77 *passim*, 114, 139,
    157; localization of, 80, 89
Tumors, spinal cord, 14, 99

Uncertainty, 26, 64–66, 97, 98, 99, 106,
    110, 139, 146–47, 193, 234–35; clinical
    vs. basic, 66, 70; diagnostic, 66, 67,
    68, 73–76, 77, 87, 93, 95; organiza-
    tional and political, 66, 67–68, 77–82,
    93, 94; taxonomic, 67, 68–73, 87, 93,
    95; technical, 67, 68, 82–85, 93, 94
Unfalsifiability, 63–65, 112
University College, London, 48, 56;
    University College Hospital, 89
University of London, 41

Validity, 107–8. *See also* Robustness
Victoria Street Society, 56. *See also* Anti-
    vivisection
Vocabularies of realism, 88–89

Wasserman test, 74
Welfare, medical, 42
Wernicke's area, 67
West Riding Pauper Lunatic Asylum, 31,
    32, 49–50, 57, 90
Work, 108–10, 187, 196–98, 233; scientific
    theories as, 1–3, 14–19, 60; and uncer-
    tainty, 63–67
Workarounds, 25
World War I, 178–79
World War II, 185

York Medical School, 164